Back Care Basics

Back Care Basics

A Doctor's Gentle Yoga Program for Back and Neck Pain Relief

By Mary Pullig Schatz, M.D.

Foreword by William Connor, M.D.
Preface by B.K.S. Iyengar

Rodmell Press
Berkeley, California
1992

First Edition
Printed in the United States of America
02   01   00   99   98   9   10   11   12   13

Library of Congress Catalog Card Number: 91-78206
ISBN 0-9627138-2-1 (softcover)
ISBN 0-9627138-5-6 (hardcover)

Anne Cushman
Editor

Andrea DuFlon
Designer

Fred Stimson
Cover Photographer

Clark Thomas/Nashville
Photographer

J. William Myers
Illustrator

Archetype Typography
Typography

McNaughton & Gunn, Inc.
Lithographer

Text set in Simoncini Garamond

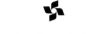

This book is dedicated

        To my father, Richard Murphy Pullig, M.D., who gave me a thirst for knowledge, an appreciation of the joy of learning, and his personal example of helping those in pain.
        To my yoga teacher, the Honorable B.K.S. Iyengar, who has unselfishly shared with me and his yoga students around the world the knowledge and experience he has gained through fifty years of teaching back patients.
        To my husband, Walter Frederick Schatz, whose steadfast love and patient companionship have helped make this book a reality.

Contents

Acknowledgments

In addition to those mentioned in the dedication, I gratefully acknowledge the following for their contributions to this work:

The dedicated men and women who were my teachers and mentors at Vanderbilt University School of Medicine and Louisiana State University School of Medicine, for giving me the Western medical background through which I could understand and appreciate the therapeutic efficacy of yoga;

My patients and students, for helping me learn to teach and to recognize the importance of the therapeutic transformations that yoga can bring about;

Anne Cushman, for her editorial professionalism, her devotion to yoga, and her gentle ways;

Carol Nelson and François Raoult for their enthusiasm and their tireless energy during long photo shoots;

Clark Thomas for his photographic expertise, his commitment to excellence, and his creative talent;

Bill Myers for his beautiful and informative drawings;

Lynne Denny for her swift and accurate secretarial support;

Betty Larson for her well-educated knees;

Donna Gurchiek for her radiant pregnant presence;

Susan Underwood, P.T., for her positive suggestions about the manuscript;

Judith Lasater, Ph.D., R.P.T., for starting me on the road to postural improvement;

Linda Cogozzo and Donald Moyer, my publishers, for their vision and tenacity in bringing this book to fruition.

Foreword

Yoga, which means "union" or "harmony," is both a philosophical system and a science whose goal is the attainment of self-awareness. With its beginnings enshrouded in the prehistory of India, evidence of yoga practices has been found in the Indus Valley civilization of 2,000 to 4,000 B.C.E. Although ancient, yoga is not outdated—it has value for the modern world. Yoga offers us the opportunity to deepen our self-understanding through physical movement, breathing, and meditation. The medical applications of yoga are numerous: It can help those with heart disease, high blood pressure, asthma, musculoskeletal problems, and, in particular, with the prevention and treatment of back pain.

The human back reflects acutely and chronically the disharmonies of our sedentary Western lifstyle. Back problems are a major health problem in our culture. They are responsible for the disability and pain of millions of Americans, and account for a large share of the health-care dollar. Dr. Mary Schatz provides us with a solution to our modern dilemma in *Back Care Basics*. She brings to her book both unusual and splendid qualifications. Dr. Schatz is a board-certified pathologist as well as chief of her hospital's medical staff in Nashville, Tennessee. She is, therefore, well-grounded in her understanding of the pathology of the diseased back. More important, she herself suffered from back pain and learned, through yoga, how to correct the problem and restore herself to good health. In this process, she studied with master yoga teacher B.K.S. Iyengar of Pune, India, who taught her how to modify traditional yoga poses to make them safer to practice during times of acute back distress. *Back Care Basics* reflects Dr. Schatz's many years of experience in applying the principles of yoga patients with back pain. She has indeed become a specialist.

I can empathize with Dr. Schatz's experience since my own life has been enriched by my four years of yoga study. My chronic hip pain, which limited my hiking considerably, has completely disappeared with daily yoga exercises. My outlook has also changed as my body, mind, and spirit become more united in purpose and achievement.

Back Care Basics is an important book for the medical profession to consider most carefully, as it is for those with back problems to integrate into their daily lives. More and more medical practitioners are finding that yoga can benefit their patients. I regularly refer my patients with coronary heart disease, obesity, and musculoskeletal problems to qualified yoga teachers, and they are encouraged with the results. Dr. Schatz has done us all a tremendous service in bringing this time-honored system of healing to our attention.

William Connor, M.D.
Professor and Head of Clinical Nutrition
Department of Medicine,
Oregon Health Sciences University
January, 1992

Preface

In *Back Care Basics,* Mary Pullig Schatz, M.D., helps to guide and educate those suffering with back pain. While explaining back problems from the viewpoint of Western medicine, she offers a comprehensive approach to self-care and healing using the ancient science of yoga.

Yoga develops the health of the body and the clarity of the mind. It also has therapeutic value, providing ways of preventing and curing diseases. Yoga enables the various parts of the body to function in harmony, keeps the cellular system healthy, and improves circulation and respiration—the main vehicles of health.

Dr. Schatz has demonstrated the efficacy of yoga by blending the thoughts of the West with those of the East. She has described the construction of the spinal column with its vertebrae and its protecting muscles in a clear and simple way, so that all can easily understand its functioning. She has given correct cautions to observe while exercising and stresses the importance of rehabilitation after injury and surgery. Her well-defined emphasis on alignment is beautiful.

I hope that *Back Care Basics* will encourage other health-care professionals to study alternative approaches to healing back pain. I am happy to have contributed to Dr. Schatz's book. If it helps suffering people, as well as those who care for them, I shall feel even more delighted for having participated in its creation.

B.K.S. Iyengar
Pune, India
January, 1992

✤ Begin with Caution

        This book is designed to help those with pain from chronic musculoskeletal back and neck strain, spinal arthritis, osteoporosis, premenstrual syndrome, pregnancy, and scoliosis. The information contained in this book is not intended as a substitute for medical treatment.

        Do not begin practicing the exercises in this book until you have studied Chapters 1 through 4 of the book, and have obtained a thorough evaluation of your condition and advice about the exercises from a qualified health-care professional who is familiar with them.

        Consult your health-care advisor:

- If you experience a worsening in severity or duration of pain after beginning this program
- If pain persists even when you are lying down in one of the Relaxation poses
- If headache, vomiting, or fever develops in association with back pain
- If back pain is associated with loss of bladder or bowel control
- If one or both legs or arms develop weakness or numbness

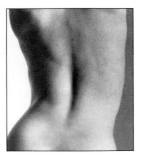

One

Yoga: The Way Back to Health

*T*his book outlines a safe, effective, low-cost approach to back rehabilitation without drugs or surgery. You'll learn a simple and practical system to heal your back, restructure your body, and cope with stress. You'll learn how your daily activities may be hurting your back and how to modify them to prevent pain and injury. You'll become more sensitive to early warning signs of an impending "back attack" and learn what to do to ward it off. Most important, you'll learn a fitness program based on a philosophy that encourages both positive health practices and a positive outlook.

No matter how serious your back problem is, rehabilitation and progress toward recovery are quite possible. If you have chronic back pain, there is more to your future than simply "learning to live with it." You can regain control of your life and free yourself from pain and disability.

Each person's spine is unique. Back exercises must be specifically tailored to *your* flexibility, strength, and habitual posture. If your back pain is related to pregnancy or your menstrual cycle, you must care for your back differently from someone whose pain is due to scoliosis or osteoporosis. A generic set of exercises may give you some relief, but a complete plan that takes into account your special circumstances has a much better chance of long-term success.

This book teaches you how to create your own personalized recovery program. You'll learn how to assess your posture, strength, and flexibility and determine how these factors affect your back. You'll learn how to adjust each exercise to make it more comfortable and effective. You'll learn how to change your exercise routine as you progress, so you continue to gain strength, flexibility, and confidence. You'll learn powerful, effective stress management and relaxation techniques.

Although the book focuses on the back, those with neck pain will find it beneficial as well. As they relax, strengthen, and realign the back, these exercises will also relieve the biomechanical imbalances that place the neck at risk.

This program is based on my own personal back recovery and my experience of over thirteen years of working with patients and yoga students with chronic back and neck pain. Its origins lie in the ancient art of hatha yoga, as refined by one of the most influential hatha yoga teachers of modern times, B.K.S. Iyengar.

What Is Yoga?

Because yoga has its roots in the Hindu culture of India, there is a popular misconception that yoga is a religion. Just as practice of the Japanese martial arts of karate and aikido does not require becoming a Buddhist, the practice of yoga does not require that you adopt Hinduism. Rather, yoga is nonsectarian, promoting health and harmonious living.

Hatha yoga hands down to modern culture the art of healing the physical body through the use of a highly sophisticated array of postures, movements, and breathing techniques. The exercises take each joint in the body through its full range of motion—strengthening, stretching, and balancing each part. When practiced regularly, the yoga poses and breathing techniques promote physical and mental health.

Yoga differs from other types of rehabilitative exercise in that it engages the whole person. The yoga-based relaxation techniques and stretching and strengthening exercises in this book are effective because the mind is focused in a meditative way on your movements, skin and muscle sensations, and relaxed breathing. Mind and body work together, creating a physiological and psychological environment that optimizes the potential for healing.

Like the steady drip of water that eventually transforms the shape of a stone, yoga works slowly but steadily to heal and restructure the tissues of your back and the supporting musculoskeletal system of your entire body. Simultaneously, it helps you recover from the psychological effects of pain and disability.

In hatha yoga as taught by B.K.S. Iyengar and presented in this book, students develop strength and endurance while observing biomechanically sound principles of alignment and correct movement. The yoga poses are carefully modified for each student's needs and abilities. The use of coordinated total body movements (rather than strengthening of isolated muscle groups, as in weight training) improves posture and body mechanics in daily activities. Thus the destructive cycles of pain and poor body mechanics are interrupted and reversed.

Practicing yoga postures gives you a more acute sense of body awareness, which alerts you to the earliest signs of back strain. Your new awareness also keeps you from repeating habitual movements, giving your body a chance to move and respond in new ways, and increasing the likelihood that the lessons you are learning will carry over into your everyday movements.

One of the greatest benefits of the yoga approach is that it helps combat the negative effects of pain, disability, and stress on your mind and body. Approaching these rehabilitation exercises in a self-exploratory way helps you learn about the sources of pain in your body and their connection to your feelings, emotions, experiences, and expectations. The yoga approach to exercise provides powerful skills for coping with the ups and downs of daily life.

Through yoga, you will learn flexibility, inner strength, and self-awareness. After only a few practice sessions, you'll begin to feel the positive changes in your body and your mind. As your body becomes more flexible, so will your thinking. As your muscles become stronger, so will your inner power. In learning to care for your back, you will learn to care for yourself better in every aspect of your life.

How To Use This Book

I know you're eager to begin your yoga program, but please refrain from skipping directly to the exercise chapters. The information and insights you will gain from the next three chapters ("Understanding Your Back," "Moving Again After Injury or Surgery," and "Assessing Your Flexibility and Alignment") are crucial to the success of this program. From these chapters, you will learn what to focus on in the "practice" chapters to follow.

After you have used Chapter 4 to assess your flexibility and alignment, take this book to your doctor or back-care therapist and discuss the exercises you plan to do. Ask your back-care professional for guidance before you begin exercising. If you have severe osteoporosis, be sure to consult your doctor before beginning this or any other exercise program.

Chapters 5 through 7 build sequentially on each other, starting with poses to rest and relax your back in Chapter 5, "Relaxation Techniques," and followed by beginning postural correction in Chapter 6, "Home Base Poses." Once the Home Base and Relaxation poses are old friends, turn to the Moving On poses in Chapter 7 to gain strength and endurance. At the end of each chapter are suggested routines to get you started. To use this program to your best advantage, it is best to stop doing your old exercises, if you were practicing any. Give yourself an entirely fresh start with yoga.

It's a good idea to read Chapters 12 and 13 ("The Yoga of Daily Living" and "Exercising Safely") early in your exploration of this book. From them you will learn how your back can be placed at risk during certain sports and daily activities. You will come to

1.1

Goal Diary

Date	Goal	Date Goal Achieved
4.1.92	To sit through a movie at the theater without pain.	9.6.92 Hooray!!

1.2

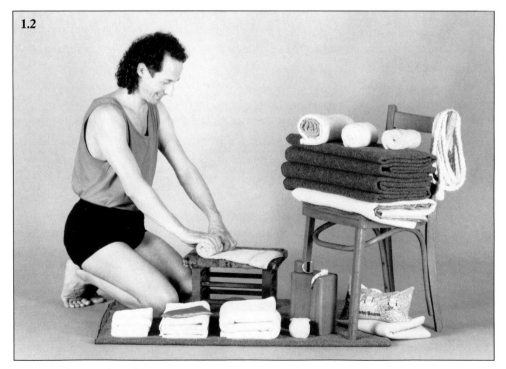

1.1 **Goal Diary, Sample Entry**
1.2 **Yoga Props**

understand the special demands these activities place on your back, and you will learn to move more safely.

If you have a specific back problem such as scoliosis, a rounded upper back, or sacroiliac dysfunction, use the chapters that focus on these problems (Chapters 8 through 10) in conjunction with Chapters 5 through 7. Chapter 13, "A Woman's Back," deals with the special problems related to pregnancy and motherhood, as well as with back pain caused by premenstrual syndrome, endometriosis, and osteoporosis.

Use the Goal Diary pages in the Appendix at the back of the book to chronicle your progress toward recovery. (See a sample entry in Figure 1.1.) Choose a few small short-term goals and a few long-term goals. What would you like most to be able to do again? Sit through a movie? Work eight hours? Walk a mile? Think positively. Set attainable goals. Visualize yourself having already attained them.

The key to persevering is knowing that you can successfully learn to manage the pain and decrease the likelihood of its recurrence. With steady work, pain can become a thing of the past. Little by little, you will change your movement patterns and rehabilitate your posture and your back. Little by little, your back attacks will become milder and less frequent.

Props for Yoga Practice

In the exercises presented in this book, various household items are used to help you modify the yoga poses for your own individual needs. These yoga props range from books and blankets to doorknobs, tables, and walls. Folded or rolled towels are used in many reclining poses to support and encourage the natural curves of the spine. Many poses also require blankets. Wool or heavy cotton blankets work best—thermal and fluffy acrylic blankets are too soft and compressible to provide firm, reliable support. Chairs are sometimes used to enable you to practice poses that otherwise might be too challenging.

Yoga props can also help bring greater awareness to your body. For example, when you sit, stand, or walk with a bag of dried beans or rice on your head, you become aware of how to maintain an erect posture.

Perhaps the most important benefit of the props is to help you practice without fear of slipping or falling. Removing the element of fear allows you to concentrate on performing the poses to the best of your ability. Avoid practicing on carpeted floors, as they will allow your feet to slip in the standing poses. A nonskid surface such as a linoleum or hardwood floor is very important. If you don't have a nonskid floor, a nonskid yoga mat (see Resources) can provide safe footing for standing poses as well as comfortable padding for kneeling and reclining poses.

Figure 1.2 shows some of the props you will need in using this book:

- beanbag (or sandbag, or bag of dried rice)
- belt (cotton webbed with D-ring buckle)
- blankets (or yoga bolsters)
- cans of soda or peas
- chair (sturdy with flat seat)
- eyebag (a rice-filled cloth bag for covering the eyes) or a folded facecloth
- nonskid mat (or other nonskid surface such as linoleum or wood)
- rope (cotton)
- socks
- stool
- towels
- wooden block (or hardcover books)

In addition, you will need a doorway, a door and doorknob, a table, and a wall.

Yoga Classes and Yoga Teachers

For the early stages of back rehabilitation, working with this book on your own or privately with a trained yoga teacher is probably safest, as people tend to overdo when first starting a class. If possible, work with a yoga teacher experienced in using yoga for the rehabilitation of back injuries. After working privately for some time with this teacher, you may want to join a class for beginners. If you can't find a teacher to work with privately, practice the Relaxation, Home Base, and Moving On poses given in Chapters 5, 6, and 7, and practice the yoga of daily living described in Chapter 12. Then consider joining a beginning class.

Choose a yoga teacher with care. Before participating, observe a class. Is the class small enough that everyone can move comfortably and get individual attention? Does the teacher observe each student in each pose? Does the teacher make individualized adjustments and corrections? Are the poses modified for the limitations and special needs of students? Do you like the way the teacher presents the material and leads the class? Does it look fun and enjoyable?

To participate safely in a class, you need a teacher who can modify poses for your requirements. It helps if the teacher has had experience with students with back challenges. Ask.

A yoga teaching certificate does not necessarily mean the teacher is qualified. Some certificates are given for attending yoga courses of only a few weeks, and many teachers receive little or no training in assessing flexibility, evaluating alignment, or adjusting poses so everyone can perform them safely. In contrast, an Iyengar-style yoga teacher's training usually includes intensive study of anatomy, physiology, yoga philosophy, and modification of poses to meet individual needs. See Resources for how to obtain information about qualified yoga teachers in North America.

There is a wealth of advice and material in this book, enough to keep you busy for several years—so don't be intimidated by the enormity of it all. It's not necessary to follow the routines at the end of each chapter item by item. If you don't have much time or you're not in the mood to practice, just do *one* exercise. (That may feel so good that you'll decide to do one or two more!) Browse through the Relaxation and Home Base poses, choose one or two poses that look like they would feel good, and start there. Just doing one pose every day is a step in the right direction. Don't let a worthy, but perhaps unrealistic, goal of practicing a certain length of time every day become a barrier to practicing at all.

The important thing is to get started down the road back to health. This book is your map.

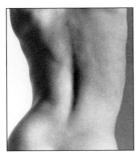

Two

Understanding Your Back

*T*o heal your back, you must understand it. Back pain results from a complex combination of factors, including posture, congenital disorders, and attitudes toward life. Viewing your pain as an illness isolated from the rest of your life may keep you from changing habits that may be perpetuating it.

Back problems do not occur in a vacuum. The spine is not an isolated body part. For a therapeutic approach to chronic back or neck strain to succeed, the spine must be seen as an integral component of a whole human being.

The state of your back is influenced by:

- Your genetic heritage
- Your home, work, transportation, play, family, and community
- Your hopes, dreams, abilities, triumphs, and tragedies
- Nutrition, body weight, and fat distribution
- Prescription and "recreational" drugs

Each of these can contribute positively or negatively to your health and the health of your back. To be successful, back care must take into account your whole being.

Your whole body affects your back. The mechanical function of your spine affects and is affected by the alignment, flexibility, and strength of many parts of your body, including:

- Foot, knee, and leg alignment
- Muscle strength of legs, buttocks, back, and abdominal wall
- Abdominal protrusion (as with a beer belly or pregnancy)
- Hip flexibility
- The position of the pelvis (tilted forward, back, or to either side)
- The shape and flexibility of the lumbar (lower back) spinal curve
- The shape and flexibility of the thoracic (upper back) spinal curve
- Shoulder carriage and the mobility of the arms at the shoulder joints
- The shape of the cervical (neck) spinal curve
- The position of the head in relation to the shoulders

For example, if your shoulder joints can't move freely, you will compensate by overarching your lower back when you reach overhead. Misalignments of your feet, knees, and legs (for example, pigeon toes, flat feet, and leg-length differences) are transferred upward, distorting your pelvis and spine. If your head is held forward of your shoulders, the muscles of your neck and upper back must overwork, creating neck pain and tension headaches.

Your whole day also affects your back. Every activity has the potential to be either therapeutic or harmful. Carefully observe the effect of everything you do, including sleep, work, driving, household chores, sports, and leisure activities such as reading and watching television (see Chapter 12, "The Yoga of Daily Living").

To be most effective, back care must not be confined to exercise time, but incorporated into a new way of life. Consider someone whose back pain is related to poor posture and body mechanics while at work (eight hours), commuting (two hours), sleeping (eight hours), and watching television (two hours). An hour of therapeutic exercise can't make up for twenty hours of destructive movement patterns.

Spinal Anatomy and Function

To begin to understand the sources of your particular back problem, it helps to understand the anatomy of the spine.

The spine is a series of intricately interlocking spool-shaped bones called *vertebrae,* supported by a complex system of muscles and ligaments. The hollow spinal canal, formed by the bony arches protruding from the back of each vertebra, protects the nerve tissue of the spinal cord.

The arms, legs, and chest all attach to the spine, via the shoulder girdle, pelvis, and ribs. The weight of the head is perched on the end of the spine. Therefore, the spine affects and is affected by every movement your body makes. For example, if the head is not properly balanced, the natural curve of the neck becomes distorted. If the arms or legs don't have a full range of motion, the spine must compensate by extra bending and twisting. Conversely, if the spine is not functioning properly, the arms, legs, and head can't move freely either. And without proper spinal alignment, the internal organs will be compressed.

The natural curves of the spine are vitally important, allowing it to act as a shock absorber during the jolts of walking, running, and sitting in a moving vehicle. The curves give the spine a strength and resilience many times that of a straight and rigid column. As an analogy, consider the difference in shock-absorbing capacity between a metal spring and a rigid pole. If you slam the end of a pole onto a hard surface, you will feel an uncomfortable jarring impact. But if you do the same thing with a coiled spring of the same material, the force will be absorbed by the spring, rather than transmitted to your body.

Viewed from the side, the curves of the spine are (Figure 2.1):

- Cervical (neck): convex in front
- Thoracic (upper back): convex behind
- Lumbar (lower back): convex in front

These normal curves lie in the front-to-back plane of the body. (Abnormal side-to-side curvature, or *scoliosis*, is discussed later.) Too much or too little curve in any of these areas can lead to dysfunction, pain, and disease.

Vertebrae

The lumbar vertebrae are massive (approximately two inches in diameter), reflecting their weight-bearing role. The cervical vertebrae are smaller, since they must support only the head. The bodies of the vertebrae are solid, roughly cylindrical blocks of bone that stack on one another, separated by the intervertebral discs (Figure 2.2). To the rear of each vertebral body, bony projections extend back from each side to form the *neural arches* that make up the spinal canal, which protects the spinal cord. The muscles that bend and rotate the spine are attached to these bony projections (which are called the *spinous* and *transverse processes*).

At the end of each of the transverse processes is a flat surface called a *facet*, which is similar to one of the facets of a cut gem (Figure 2.3). The facets of one vertebra form joints (*facet joints*) with the facets of the vertebrae above and below. The slant of the facet surfaces determines the directions the vertebrae can move. Back or neck pain identical to that caused by a herniated intervertebral disc can be caused by abnormalities (such as arthritis) in the facet joints.

Intervertebral Discs

Understanding disc function and dysfunction—the source of a great deal of back pain—is easy once you comprehend disc structure.

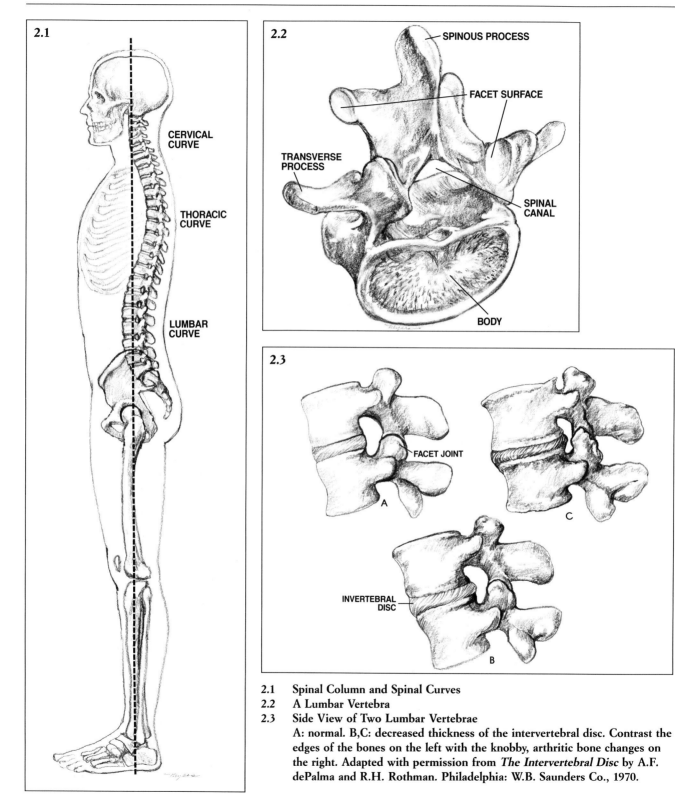

2.1   Spinal Column and Spinal Curves
2.2   A Lumbar Vertebra
2.3   Side View of Two Lumbar Vertebrae
      A: normal. B,C: decreased thickness of the intervertebral disc. Contrast the
      edges of the bones on the left with the knobby, arthritic bone changes on
      the right. Adapted with permission from *The Intervertebral Disc* by A.F.
      dePalma and R.H. Rothman. Philadelphia: W.B. Saunders Co., 1970.

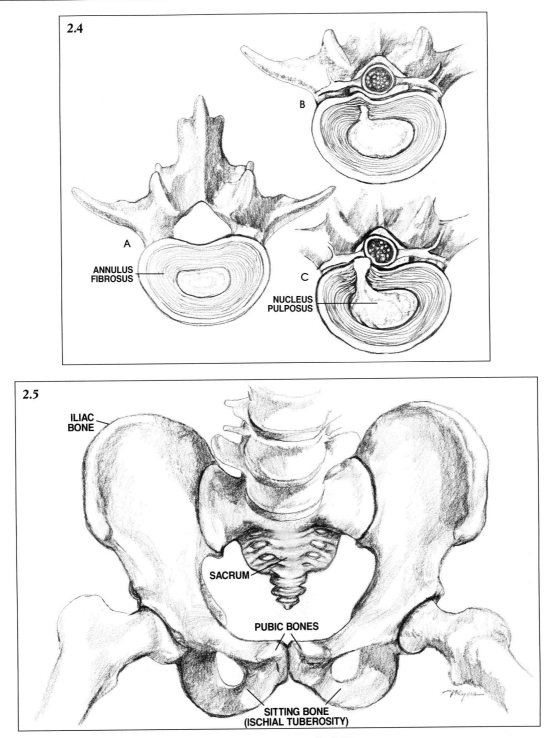

2.4 A: Normal, B: Bulging, and C: Herniating Intervertebral Discs
Adapted with permission from *The Invertebral Disc* by A.F. dePalma and R.H. Rothman.
Philadelpha: W.B. Saunders Co., 1970.

2.5 Sacrum and Pelvis

Discs are thick pads of cartilage that separate adjacent vertebrae. Together, they make up one-fourth of the length of the vertebral column. The discs serve as shock absorbers and allow greater motion between the vertebrae than would be possible if the bones were in direct contact with each other. Most important, they distribute weight over a large surface when the spine bends. When discs degenerate, this weight becomes concentrated on the edges of the vertebrae, resulting in bone spurs.

Discs are composed of a special form of cartilage called *fibrocartilage*, a composite of cartilage and fibrous tissue. The outer edge, formed of interwoven rings of very strong fibrocartilage, is called the *annulus fibrosus*. The center of the disc, called the *nucleus pulposus*, is a soft, pulpy, gelatin-like substance. If the tough outer ring weakens or tears, the inner gel can bulge or extrude (*herniate*) through it, painfully pressing against the spinal nerves (Figure 2.4).

The disc acquires its nourishment through the fluid-attracting and fluid-absorbing qualities of the gel-like nucleus pulposus. With no blood supply of its own, the disc is dependent on sponge action for attracting and absorbing nutrients from adjacent tissues. During nonweight-bearing rest, the discs expand as they soak up fluid, increasing the length of the spine by as much as one inch overnight. In weight-bearing activity, this fluid is squeezed back into the adjacent soft tissues and vertebrae, to be replaced by fresh fluid during the next rest period. If these normal healing mechanisms are inhibited by poor posture and loss of flexibility, the discs become thin, brittle, and easily injured. This condition, called *degenerative disc disease*, can lead to bulging or herniated discs. The movement principles of therapeutic yoga—"spreading" (creating space in an area), "soaking" (allowing blood and fluids to bathe and cleanse an area), and "squeezing" (compressing fluids out of an area)—use the physiology of the disc to help in healing.

Spinal Cord and Nerve Roots

Literally an extension of the brain, the spinal cord is a bundle of nerves that travels down through the spinal canal, which is formed by a series of arches in the vertebrae (the *neural arches,* discussed earlier). When a nerve branches off of the cord, it exits the spinal column via and *intervertebral foramen* (a hole between two vertebrae). At this exit point, the nerve is vulnerable to compression by a bulging or herniated intervertebral disc.

Sacrum and Pelvis

The pelvis is a funnel-shaped group of relatively flat bones, higher in the back than in the front. Because the joints between the bones of the pelvis allow very little motion, the pelvis effectively functions as a single bone (Figure 2.5). The end of the spinal column (the tailbone and the flat, triangular bone called the *sacrum*, which is formed by the fusion of the last five vertebrae) forms part of the back wall of the pelvis, and the upper ends of the thigh bones insert into sockets in its side walls. Thus, the pelvis joins the spine to the legs.

Because the end of the spine (the sacrum) forms part of the pelvic funnel, the position of the pelvis has profound effects on the lumbar curve. You can experience this connection by performing this simple exercise: Sit on a firm chair with a flat seat. Tilt your pelvis forward so your navel moves forward toward your knees and your tailbone moves up and back. With your hands on your back, feel how this motion increases the lumbar curve to a more swaybacked position. Now tilt your pelvis backward by tucking your tailbone and moving your navel toward your spine. Notice how your lumbar spine flattens.

Muscles That Act on the Spine

The bony structures of the spine and pelvis are supported and moved by many different muscles, whose condition can profoundly affect the state of your lower back. If any of these muscles are tight or weak, they can create or worsen back pain.

Running parallel to your spine are the *paraspinal* muscles, deep muscles of the back that function as guy wires to support the spine in the upright position (Figure 2.6). (To feel the paraspinals, put your hand on your back at waist level. The slight bulges you feel on either side of the spine are formed by the paraspinal muscles.) The paraspinals rotate the spine, bend it backward and sideways, and influence posture by helping create and maintain the proper spinal curves. If the paraspinals are too tight, they contribute to a swayback. If they are too stretched out, they contribute to a flat back. If they are overworked, they can go into painful spasms. Yoga helps maintain back health by both stretching and strengthening the paraspinals.

The lower back is also significantly influenced by three sets of muscles that attach to the pelvis or the lumbar vertebrae: the hip flexors (which raise the thigh toward the chest), the abdominals, and the hamstrings (the long muscles on the back of the thigh) (Figure 2.7). By altering the forward or backward tilt of the pelvis, these muscles can increase or decrease the lumbar curve. For example, because the hip flexors attach to the front of the pelvis, tight hip flexors will tilt the pelvis forward, creating a swayback. Tight hamstrings will tilt the pelvis backward, creating a flat back. Weak abdominal muscles will allow the pelvis to drop forward and will fail to support the lumbar spine from the front. You will learn more about these muscles and how they function in Chapter 4, "Assessing Your Flexibility and Alignment."

Your Neck and Your Back

Since it is actually a part of the spine, your neck can be affected by many of the same conditions that affect your back, including muscle strain, degenerative disc disease, and arthritis. When they are chronically stressed, the intervertebral discs in the neck can also bulge or herniate. A herniated cervical disc can cause pain, weakness, or numbness in the shoulder, arm, or hand.

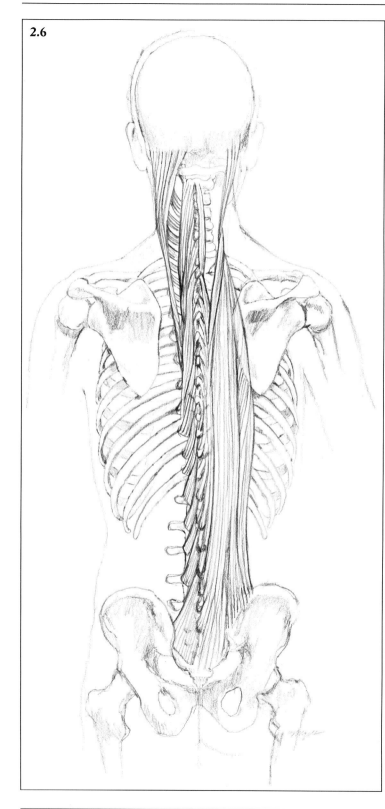

2.6

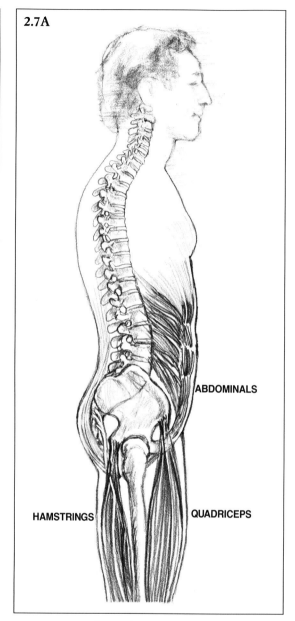

2.7A

ABDOMINALS

HAMSTRINGS

QUADRICEPS

2.6   **Paraspinal Muscles**
2.7A **Muscles That Affect the Lower Back Curve and the Tilt of the Pelvis. The abdominal muscles support the spine from the front, and can pull the pubic bone up to flatten the lower back or let the pelvis drop down thereby creating sway-back. The quadriceps, part of the hip flexor group, can contribute to swayback by pulling the front sides of the pelvis down. The hamstrings can contribute to a flat lumbar curve if they are short and tight.**

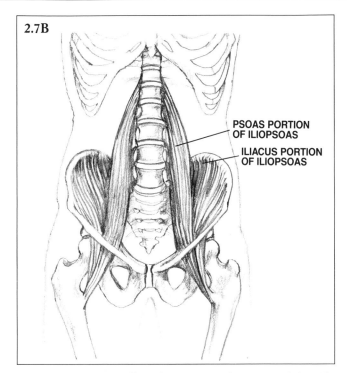

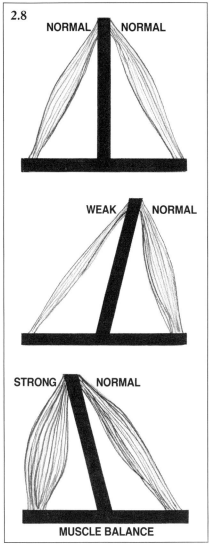

2.7B Muscles That Affect the Lower Back Curve and the Tilt of the Pelvis. The iliopsoas muscles, part of the hip flexor group, can contribute to swayback by pulling the lumbar vertebrae and the flared part of the back of the pelvis forward and down.

2.8 Muscle Balance. When muscles acting on both sides of a joint are well-balanced, the joint is kept in good alignment. If the muscles are unbalanced, proper joint movement is compromised and the joint is at risk for injury. Adapted with permission from *Applied Kinesiology, Volume 1: Basic Procedures and Muscle Testing* by D.W. Walther. Pueblo, Colo.: Systems D.C., 1981.

Posture and Back Pain

Once you understand the anatomy of the spinal column, it is easy to see how every movement you make throughout the day affects the well-being of your back. A crucial step in understanding your back pain is to understand your own posture—the way you habitually hold your body. Most back problems result not from congenital bone disorders, but from poor posture or improper use of the spine. The way you stand, the way you sit, the way you move, the way you pick up and carry objects—all these things have the potential to help or hurt your back.

Many people permanently adopt the posture that their daily occupation encourages them to relax into. An accountant's rounded shoulders, a couch potato's slouch, and the bowed head of someone who is depressed are just a few examples of habitual postures that can lead to lower back pain. Prolonged postural imbalances can lead to more serious problems, such as degenerative disease of the intervertebral discs (including bulging discs and herniated discs), arthritis, and degeneration or deformation of the vertebrae.

Fortunately, correcting poor posture is possible. Most people understand that posture can change, but their experience of this shift is usually limited to the deterioration that occurs with age: the postural changes they see as they watch their parents, aunts, and uncles age. Most people don't understand that positive change is also possible. Posture is only partially genetically determined. It is influenced just as strongly by whom we choose to mimic as children, by our self-images during childhood and adolescence, and by traumas and injuries. Posture frequently changes for the worse; this book shows how posture can change for the better.

Imitating Role Models

Although your basic posture is dependent on the bone structure you inherited from your parents, it is also shaped by other conscious and unconscious factors. Your posture reflects both your role models and your own self-image.

One of my favorite vacation pastimes is watching the beach walkers, their backs undisguised by bulky clothes. As families stroll along the shore, I am frequently struck by the similarity in posture and gait between parents and their children, and between parents and their children, and between children and their peers. It is a heartwarming sight to observe a six-year-old boy smile up lovingly at his father and perfectly mimic the paternal beach saunter. Later that day, I might see the same child trying on the posture and gait of an older boy. Young girls round their shoulders forward to hide budding breasts.

Become aware of your role models and realize that you can choose to hold yourself differently. One of my yoga students, a young mother in her twenties, was developing neck, shoulder, and upper back problems because of her markedly rounded upper back. Because both her mother and grandmother had the same posture, she had accepted it as inevitable. As an adolescent, she had not understood that the older women's stooped posture was caused by osteoporosis, and therefore she had never permitted herself an alternative. She found it hard to begin to work on her upper back posture; she used the fact that it ran in her family as an excuse not to try and change it.

Many young girls choose such poor postural role models as the Olympic gymnasts, whose triumphantly exaggerated swaybacked stance at the end of their routines exhibits an abnormal and destructive posture in a setting associated with health and vigor. (Gymnasts have a high incidence of fractures of the lumbar spine and vertebral dislocation due to the trauma they inflict on the lumbar vertebrae.) Similarly, boys and men often imitate the rounded shoulders and forward head of professional and collegiate basketball players as they slump on the sidelines.

Imitating someone else's stance can be positive if the person you choose to imitate has good posture. I remember the stately, regal feeling I experienced when I decided to try on the posture and gait of my tall, elegant yoga teacher. Almost immediately I felt taller and more serene.

Posture and Emotion

Your mood dramatically affects your posture, and, conversely, your posture affects your mood. Take a few moments for an experiment. Remember the last time you were depressed and picture yourself going through your daily activities in this state. Remember your feelings of despair or defeat. What posture do you see in your mind's eye? Is your head bowed and your back rounded? Are your shoulders drooped? Are you holding your head in your hands?

Examine your actual posture at this moment. Has the mere thought of this past depression affected your current posture?

Now take yourself back to a period of excitement or joy. Picture the street, house, or workplace that was the setting for this happy time. See yourself moving through your daily activities. Is your face animated, smiling, laughing? Are your movements energetic? Does the posture you remember indicate openheartedness?

Observe your own posture right now. Does it more closely reflect the posture of happiness or the posture of sorrow?

You have just observed the effect of mental state on posture. Now try the effect of posture on mental state. Assume a depressed posture and gait for three to five minutes. Let your face be slack and without animation. Let your head hang forward and your shoulders slouch. Move as little as possible. Recreate the body language of lethargy.

When the time is up, examine your thoughts and feelings. Have they been affected by your posture and movements?

You are now beginning to understand—with your body as well as your mind—the influence of mind on body and body on mind. Remember these lessons as you move through the exercises in this book, many of which involve assuming positions of strength and determination. The body language of each pose or exercise sends you a positive message, just as the body language of depression sends you a negative one. Approaching the exercises with a positive state of mind will increase their effectiveness.

Selective Stretching and Strengthening

Posture is affected not only by your mental state, but by muscular strengths and weaknesses developed over time. Besides affecting your mood and body language, yoga exercises can also affect your posture in very direct, specific ways, by selectively stretching and strengthening the muscles that control it.

Each of your joints is controlled by at least two sets of muscles: the *flexors*, which bend the joint, and the *extensors*, which straighten it. In addition, a number of joints have *rotator* muscles that twist, turn, or rotate the bones. Good posture can exist only when the flexors, extensors, and rotators are in proper balance, allowing each joint to function efficiently (Figure 2.8). In a well-balanced joint, the cartilage surfaces at the ends of the bones move against each other in a way that promotes orderly repair of the joint tissues.

But often, the muscles acting upon a joint are out of balance. For example, the flexors may be tighter and shorter than the extensors, so that the joint cannot be fully straightened; or the muscles that rotate the joint in one direction may be stronger than those that rotate it the other way. These unequal forces make the joint weaker and more vulnerable. Parts of the bone surfaces bear more weight than they should. By altering the normal regenerative processes that keep joints healthy, this imbalance can cause pain and arthritis.

Many people with back or neck pain suffer from an imbalance of the flexors, extensors, and rotators of the spine, arms, and legs. With an intelligent program of stretching and strengthening, the muscle groups can be brought back into balance. In the following chapters, you will learn how to assess your own muscle group imbalances and how to safely perform exercises that can put your muscles back into balance.

As your muscle groups become more balanced, your posture will begin to change. But along with doing the exercises to balance muscle groups and realign the body, you must mentally allow yourself to have an improved posture. Your mental concepts of who you are and what you look like are translated into the way you carry your body. If you keep the same self-image as you had when your back pain began, these exercises will be of limited value.

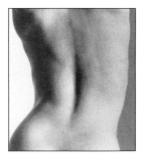

Three

Moving Again After Injury or Surgery

*A*nyone who has experienced back pain and disability understands the fear of exercising again. Most back patients fear that any movement or exercise might cause reinjury. But without an intelligent exercise program to rehabilitate not only the back, but the entire body and the psyche, reinjury is not only likely but practically inevitable.

Although rest is often needed for several days after a spinal injury, prolonged inactivity is counterproductive. When your back or neck hurts, it is natural to seek relief by resting. But if inactivity persists for very long, the muscles that usually support the back become weak, and it becomes increasingly vulnerable to reinjury. Reinjury creates more pain, which elicits more inactivity, which causes more muscle weakness, which further predisposes you to injury. This cycle of deterioration is further accelerated by the depression that can accompany inactivity and pain.

However, you may not know how to distinguish between exercises that will help your back and exercises that will hurt it. Furthermore, you may not understand how your injury or surgery has affected your back—you may feel that something mysterious has happened "behind your back" and have only a hazy perception of what is really "back there" now. If you are recovering from injury or surgery, this chapter will give you a clearer understanding of what has happened to your back, how healing has further altered it, and how best to approach healthy moving again.

The Importance of Exercise and Good Body Mechanics

Some people feel so good after surgery or in between "back attacks" that they erroneously imagine that their problems have been cured. They think that because their problems have disappeared or been surgically corrected, they no longer need to pay attention to their backs. Without pain as a reminder, the need to care for the back recedes in the consciousness. The important thing to remember, however, is that the pain may have been cured only temporarily. The underlying problems (postural strain and muscular imbalances) remain to cause trouble in the future.

If you have had surgery, not only do the underlying problems remain, but additional postsurgical structural weaknesses have now been added, along with muscular weakness related to inactivity. Therefore it is vital that postoperative time and energy be devoted to an intelligent yoga-based exercise program and to the yoga of daily living (proper body mechanics). If, after surgical recovery, you continue with the same posture and the same ways of moving and using your body, injury will recur.

It is up to you to build yourself a healthier spine. The surgeon cannot create a new back, but you can.

Scar Tissue

Following injury, whether due to trauma or surgery, the body heals itself by producing scar tissue. The amount of scarring depends upon the extent of the injury or surgery. For example, in surgery that consists only of inserting a suction needle to extract a damaged disc, there is minimal injury to surrounding tissue. In that case the amount of scarring depends upon the severity of the injury that made the surgery necessary. However, if there has been extensive surgery (such as is required for a vertebral fusion), then there will be considerable scarring at all of the levels affected by the surgery, including muscles, ligaments, nerves, and bones. Besides specific, accidental traumas or one-time surgery, repeated small traumas can also result in scarring.

Scar tissue looks like the white fasciae and tendons you see in red meat. This connective tissue, which separates muscles and attaches muscles to bone, is the same type of tissue formed during the healing process. During this process, this connective tissue is organized into groups of stringlike collagen bundles, something like skeins of yarn. In its early stages, this collagen can be easily stretched and molded. In later stages (when the scar tissue is more than six months old), collagen becomes more resistant to stretch.

Once the collagen is formed, it begins to shorten and pull together all of the injured tissues. This action is important for bringing the edges of a wound together. Unfortunately, a nerve in the area can become entrapped in the scar. When this happens, stretching of the scar may result in painful stretching of a nerve. Because a basic characteristic of scar tissue is that it shrinks, it becomes more and more likely that an entrapped nerve will be stretched whenever the shortened scar has tension put on it.

For those who have had back injury or surgery, scarring in the muscle and soft tissue can reduce normal movement between the vertebrae. This *hypomobile* (insufficiently mobile) segment is no longer able to move naturally. The resultant increased slack in the supporting muscles and ligaments allows the segments above and below the hypomobile segment to become *hypermobile* (exessively mobile) and prone to further injury. The facet joints can also develop arthritis due to abnormally increased movement.

Because of this increased vulnerability, it is important that after injury or surgery you become finely attuned to the sensations and feelings in the areas just above and just below the injured site. You may notice that you often feel strain at one or both of these places during certain positions and movements. This is important information that will help in adjusting exercises and posture.

In the postoperative or postinjury period (after the first weeks of recovery), an intelligent exercise program can help scar tissue grow in a healthier configuration. Remember that the primary job of scar tissue is to pull the edges of the wound together and hold them securely. When it is first forming, scar tissue is easier to stretch. After six months it becomes harder (although not impossible) to increase the length of a scar. Thus, as soon as you can stretch and move the site of the operation or injury (your doctor will tell you when), mild stretches can help the scar tissue lengthen so that it is less likely to limit movement and encroach upon nerves.

For those who have old scars, do not despair—scars can respond to stretching even after they have matured. It just takes more patience. Hold the stretches longer (at least ninety seconds), gradually working up to several minutes several times a day. Although the physical therapy literature has focused on mechanical devices that hold stretches for twenty minutes at a time, my experience with yoga stretches has shown that progress can be made with durations of five to ten minutes in stretching yoga poses.

Prolonged Bed Rest As a Cause of Back Pain

Although bed rest for one to three days is frequently prescribed for acute back pain, prolonged bed rest for any reason can actually lead to back pain. If the muscles supporting the spine are not required to work by holding the body upright in sitting and standing positions, they rapidly weaken. This muscular weakness, combined with other physiological changes due to prolonged inactivity, creates a propensity for back instability, which can lead to injury and further disability.

As if prolonged bed rest and weakness were not enough, hospitalization compounds the problem of bed rest by placing the spine in one of the most dangerous environments of all: the hospital bed! The hospital bed can make your back problem worse, because it tends to keep your spine rounded. If the head of the bed is raised for reading or watching television, you tend to slip down toward the foot of the bed. This can be alleviated by raising the knee portion of the bed. This, however, places you with the lower back rounded, which is distinctly disadvantageous. Rounding the lower back stretches the paraspinal muscles and the ligaments that support the lumbar spine. When you do emerge from the bed, the lumbar spine is weak and unstable.

To make matters worse, the thick, incompressible hospital pillow causes the head to be held far in front of the chest. This is a perfect setup for a neckache as well as a backache.

For a patient in the hospital after abdominal, thoracic, or pelvic surgery, the risk to the back is even greater. A patient quickly learns that any sensation of stretch around the operative incision site creates pain. The patient therefore maintains a hunched position to decrease tension along the incision.

Add to these postural problems the muscle weakness and postural instability caused by painkilling medication, and the likelihood for back injury is high.

To prevent back injury associated with bed rest and surgery:

- Provide proper spinal support for the natural spinal curves when sitting up in bed. (Support the lumbar and neck curves with rolled towels and place a rolled towel or pillow behind the knees, as shown in Figures 5.3–5.6 and 5.14.)
- Change position often, alternately lying on the right side, the left side, and the back.
- Be aware that the psychological effects of bed rest include boredom, irritability, and depression, so that these don't catch you by surprise and alarm you.
- Never sit straight up from a lying position. Always get out of bed slowly and carefully, by first rolling all the way onto your side and using the strength of the arms to push yourself up into a sitting position, with the legs already over the side of the bed. Sit for thirty to sixty seconds before standing, to avoid dizziness or lightheadedness.
- Exercise in bed to enhance circulation, keep muscles strong, and prevent boredom and depression. Try practicing some of the Relaxation or Home Base poses that can be done lying down, such as Supine Pelvic Tilt (Figure 6.1), Crocodile Twist (Figure 6.7), or Supine Knee-Chest Twist (Figure 6.5).

Principles of Postoperative/Postinjury Exercise Therapy

Because motivation is a key element in whether you practice an exercise program faithfully, it is important for those with postoperative/postinjury back challenges to understand the benefits of exercise and to learn the basic principles of back rehabilitation. Knowing the specific benefits to be achieved is more helpful than vaguely understanding that "exercise is good for my back." Understanding these principles will help answer the question, "What is this exercise doing for my back?"

The basic principles of postoperative/postinjury exercise therapy are as follows:

Reeducate yourself about posture and movement. You must reeducate your body, so that the same musculoskeletal imbalances that predisposed you to the original injury do not continue in this new, slightly more vulnerable situation. Learning improved ways of sitting, standing, and working can reduce the likelihood of a recurrent or new injury in the adjacent, hypermobile segment. Specific exercises and awareness lessons for better body mechanics and improved posture are presented in Chapter 12, "The Yoga of Daily Living." Every exercise and activity throughout the day should improve your posture and alignment.

Strengthen the muscles that support your back. The main muscle groups to be strengthened are the abdominals, leg muscles, and paraspinals. Strengthening of muscles is especially important if you have become weak and debilitated. If you have a weak leg from nerve damage, you must work to strengthen the remaining muscles. The leg that is not damaged must also be strengthened, as it is required to do more work.

Increase flexibility. Increasing flexibility in your shoulders and hips will decrease demands on your back. Remember that if your arms cannot be stretched fully overhead or your legs cannot be fully straightened at the hips, you will place excessive demands for movement on your lumbar spine. Flexibility is also important to allow your spine to rotate properly. The muscle groups that must be stretched to provide improved flexibility include the hip flexors (the muscles that bend the leg up toward the chest), the hamstring muscles (the back thigh muscles), and the paraspinals (the muscles on either side of the spine).

Increase leg and buttock strength for proper lifting. From a biomechanical standpoint, lifting well requires more than just strong arms or a strong back. It also requires strength and flexibility of the legs and hips. As you will learn in Chapter 12, "The Yoga of Daily Living," lifting a heavy load well requires a fair amount of flexibility in the hips, knees, and ankles in order to get close enough to the load to lift it with your legs instead of your back. Of course, arm strength is needed to hug the load close to your body. The lifting of the load, however, is done by the large, strong muscles of the buttocks and legs. Increasing the strength and flexibility of these areas will decrease the demands on your back during lifting.

Refrain from smoking. Smoking decreases blood circulation to the discs. Disc nutrition is decreased by as much as thirty percent to forty percent by smoking for twenty to thirty minutes. It can take as long as two hours for disc circulation to return to normal after smoking.

Gain pain relief through exercise. The body produces its own internal tranquilizers and painkillers, called "endorphins." It has been shown that the spinal fluid of those with chronic back pain has a decreased level of endorphins. It has also been shown that spinal fluid endorphins can be increased by exercise that activates large muscle groups. An increase in spinal fluid endorphins will decrease your sensitivity to pain. As you perform the exercises in this book, you can feel confident that you will experience a pain-reducing effect, in addition to the long-term benefits of postural correction, improved body mechanics, and improved mental outlook.

Learn awareness of the early warning signs. Become intimately acquainted with your "signal spot," the place that hurts when your back first begins bothering you. Your spot may be at the segment above or below the level of your surgery or injury. Frequently it will feel strain or pain before your back "goes out." Become very familiar with your signal spot. How does it feel? Reach back and touch it. See if you can visualize the bones, the muscles, and any scar tissue that might be there. As you move through the exercises, focus on this image of your spot. Notice how your signal spot changes as it responds to the healing effects of the exercises.

What are some of the early warning signs? These vary immensely from one person to another, but are usually fairly constant for each individual. It may be a slight feeling of discomfort or warmth at your signal spot. It may be a feeling of strain or general discomfort in your upper or lower back. You may notice difficulty getting out of a soft chair. You may find your hand going to your signal spot to give it support during difficult movements. An early warning sign may be muscle soreness or tenderness over your spot or a dull ache of the muscles around it. Increasing your ability to perceive and respond to subtle signals is natural biofeedback. Act upon these caution signals by using poses from Chapter 5, "Relaxation Techniques," and by decreasing back-challenging activity for a while until things settle down.

Be your own personal therapist using natural biofeedback. You know more (or can learn more) about your own back and its responses to challenges than anyone else, including your doctor. Only you can use your own natural biofeedback to feel and respond to the earliest warning signs of impending pain in order to avoid a full-blown back attack. Only you can feel the subtle changes that correction of posture and improvement of body mechanics can make in the way your back and neck feel. By the time you get to your health-care professional with a complaint of pain, it is usually too late to prevent major discomfort.

By practicing the exercises and techniques outlined in this book, you can become finely attuned to the early warning signals from the doctor within. You can learn to discriminate between prepain and pain. You can learn what to do at the first signals of prepain and thereby avoid the true disability that accompany a full-blown attack.

Understanding and Working with Your Pain

In my work with back patients, many of whom have had multiple surgical procedures, I have often been struck by their fear of exercise. Most of them have had unpleasant, painful experiences with the "no pain, no gain" approach to exercise, and at first don't realize that they can adapt exercises so there is little or no pain. Most of them feel that they hurt all over and that practically everything they do causes them pain. It is helpful for them to begin to realize that the pain is not constant, to become aware of the conditions existing when they hurt, and to be able to pinpoint exactly where and how they hurt. Once they gain this knowledge, they are able to modify their exercises and learn more body awareness to prevent additional injury.

Those who have had back injuries or surgery must learn to distinguish among the various types of sensations that may be perceived as pain. These include *muscle stretch sensation, muscle overstretch pain, radiating nerve pain* (shooting, burning pain like an electric shock), *scar stretch pain,* and *postexercise pain.*

Any movement or position that creates numbness or the sharp electric shock of nerve pain should be modified so the basic movement can be performed without creating either of these sensations. This approach may be new for those who have been told to cease doing an exercise that created numbness or pain, as well as for those from the "no pain, no gain" school of thought. Deleting painful exercises can result in the elimination of some of the exercises that could be most beneficial if properly adjusted for your needs. But persisting with an exercise, hoping to work through the pain, is counterproductive. Numbness, nerve pain, or the pain of muscle overstretching are signals of wrong movement. When these sensations are created, the body reacts by tensing muscles, which can create more pain and further imbalances.

When performing stretching exercises, you must learn to play the edge between the sensation of *muscle stretch* and the pain of *muscle overstretch*. Your limits will vary from day to day and from one side of the body to the other. If a stretch feels painful, decrease the intensity of the stretch to a tolerable level. By "tolerable," I don't mean that you can stand it if you grit your teeth, but rather that you can relax into the position and quietly allow the muscles to stretch and lengthen. The sensation of a muscle stretch should be a pleasant pulling and lengthening. Remember that a stretch must be held fifteen to twenty seconds in order for the muscle to get the message to relax and lengthen.

Radiating nerve pain is due to nerve compression, often by a herniated intervertebral disc, and is felt along the pathway of the nerve, all the way to the periphery of the body. Often constant, this pain indicates that the nerve is being injured, usually by a herniated disc being pressed onto it. In what is known as *referred pain*, the pain is not felt along the entire length of the nerve, but is only perceived in the periphery of the body as buttock, hip, thigh, knee, lower leg, or foot pain (even though the actual source of the pain may be nerve compression in the lower back). If there is nerve compression in the neck, there can be pain or numbness in the shoulder, arm, hands, or fingers.

Nerve pain may also be associated with weakness in the muscles controlled by the injured or irritated nerve and by numbness in the affected area. In lumbar disc disease, the muscle weakness sometimes manifests as foot dragging or stumbling. If nerve compression is long-lasting, it may cause shrinkage of calf, thigh, or buttock muscles and permanent nerve damage. In cervical disc disease, the hand and arm can be affected. *Do not create nerve pain during your exercises.* If such pain persists despite modification of the poses as suggested, check with your doctor.

Scar stretch pain is due to stretching of shortened connective tissues around a previously injured vertebral segment. This is a necessary pain. When shortened connective tissues are stretched properly, no injury results. This type of pain usually does not radiate into the buttock or down the leg, but is confined to the scarred tissues adjacent to the spine. (There may, however, be an occasional brief radiation of pain if a nerve is trapped in the scar tissue.) Scar stretch pain is not constant, but appears in body positions that stretch the scar and disappears when that position is released. You must learn to play the edge of scar stretch pain so tearing of the soft tissues does not occur, yet sufficient stretch is placed on the shortened connective tissues to begin to create increased length. Persistent, repeated, gentle stretches held for at least two to four minutes at a time is necessary for remodeling of mature scar (scar older than six months) and shortened connective tissues.

Scar stretch pain, nerve pain, and muscle overstretch are of short duration and end as soon as the stretch is released or the incorrect action is altered. Another type of pain, *postexercise pain*, begins after the exercise session is over and persists for several hours, usually as a dull ache. This delayed and prolonged pain after exercise is common for people who have arthritis of the spine or scarring related to longstanding problems or surgery. It must be tolerated to a point (though lessened as much as possible). A basic rule is that if pain persists for more than two to three hours after exercising, you should alter the amount, intensity, or alignment of the exercises.

Prolonged pain after exercise calls for a reevaluation of the exercise session. Was it too long? Were the individual movements done with too much intensity? Were stretches held for too long? Were some of the poses held in poor alignment?

At first it may not be apparent exactly where the problem lies. This is where a yoga teacher with a good eye for alignment is of great benefit. If you have no success in reducing pain after decreasing the intensity or duration of the poses, a yoga teacher experienced in therapeutic work can suggest ways to improve alignment (see Resources).

Pain, Fear, and the Yoga Solution

Pain is magnified and perpetuated by fear. It is, conversely, diminished by calm observation.

In any painful situation, there are two main components that determine how much pain you perceive: the basic pain and the pain that is superimposed by your reaction to the basic pain. This superimposed pain comes from the feelings of fear, helplessness, and uncertainty that are generated by the basic pain. You begin to worry: How long will the pain last? Will it stay like this or will it get worse? When will it get worse? How long will I be incapacitated? What if it never stops? Is something terrible wrong with me?

This anxiety magnifies and perpetuates the pain through the mechanisms of the stress cycle (described in more detail in Chapter 5, "Relaxation Techniques"). When pain occurs during an exercise, the automatic stress response is that muscles in the area tighten up. Pain increases. This confirms your worst fears: You're not getting better, the exercises are hurting you, and you'll never get well. You stop trying to exercise. Pain and deterioration continue. This combination of pain plus stress reaction is especially potent if you are attempting therapeutic exercise for an injury.

Yoga offers a way to transform this distressing situation. Through its natural biofeedback processes, yoga teaches you to observe and analyze painful situations from a detached viewpoint, to make adjustments and reassessments. Instead of panicking, you learn to ask yourself useful questions that can lead to a constructive solution: How was I moving when the pain started? Was it just muscle stretch sensation or was it true pain? If it was true pain, was it nerve pain or overstretch pain? If I adjust my position this way and decrease the intensity of the stretch, what happens? Can I use my breath to exhale some of this pain? Can I visualize the pain leaving my body?

As you go through this process, apparent miracles occur:

- You become separate from the pain.
- You learn that you have a choice about whether you will react to the pain and make it worse or detach, observe, and adjust the exercise so that the pain decreases.
- Fear of the worst gives way to a sense of control.
- Helplessness gives way to competence.
- The unknown cause of the pain becomes known and better understood.
- You learn how a wrong movement can cause pain and a more correct movement can diminish it.

• You learn about the power of conscious breathing and imagery to reduce pain and give you control.

Thus yoga gives you a pain-minimizing strategy that helps you teach yourself to create less and less pain.

Won't Doing Yoga Hurt My Back?

Yoga will help, not harm, your back—provided you approach it with the proper attitude. Intelligent yoga is rehabilitative. But yoga—or any other exercise—done carelessly or aggressively can be harmful.

Do not approach your yoga practice hastily or aggressively. Constant attention to breathing and alignment distinguishes yoga from calisthenics and acrobatics, making it rehabilitative for the body and the spirit. Using each pose to create inner quietness and peace will move you toward healing and rejuvenation.

But if you attempt to do yoga poses without attention to the principles of good body mechanics and proper spinal alignment, you can hurt yourself. If you have limited flexibility, you can suffer back injuries in forward bends or backbends if you do not perform them with respect for your current degree of flexibility. And if you attempt to fit your inflexible (or overly flexible) body into yoga poses as demonstrated by accomplished yoga practitioners, harm can result.

In order to change yoga from a potential danger to a rehabilitative practice, you must follow the steps outlined in this book or seek a teacher experienced in adapting yoga to rehabilitative purposes. The proper poses, done with care for alignment and adapted for your flexibility, can be the perfect rehabilitation program.

Forward bends, backbends, twists, and standing poses can be either therapeutic or detrimental for your back, depending on how well you honor the principle of maintaining normal spinal curves. The most frequently abused postures are forward bends (standing and seated) and backbends; therefore, extreme versions of these poses are not recommended as part of a back rehabilitation program and are not included in this book.

Because many back injuries occur as a result of lifting while twisting, some people fear that yoga poses in which there is spinal rotation might be injurious to those with back problems. However, the yoga twists described in this book are safe if they are done with the spine properly aligned and supported. The key to safe and therapeutic spinal twists is that they be done with the spine in its normal or neutral configuration. If you have a posture problem (such as an increased thoracic curve, inflexibility in the thoracic spine, lumbar lordosis, or a flat lumbar curve) and you encounter any problems with the twisting poses, seek the guidance of a teacher experienced in the use of Iyengar-style yoga therapy for back problems.

Whereas other physical therapy approaches emphasize either flexion (bending the spine forward) or extension (bending the spine backward), the Iyengar approach to back rehabilitation emphasizes full range of motion. Supported positions of spinal flexion ease paraspinal muscle spasm. Gentle, properly aligned spinal twists safely stretch the paraspinal muscles and increase intervertebral space and spinal mobility. Standing poses strengthen the back muscles, abdominal muscles, and legs for improved carriage, spinal support, and safe lifting. Supported backbends gently place the spine in a position of extension without the danger of lumbar compression. These elements make up the rehabilitative yoga program presented in this book.

Backsliding: What To Do If You Have Lapsed in Your Practice

After beginning this rehabilitation program, despite your best interests and best intentions, you may lapse in your yoga practice. Some people neglect exercise and stress management when things are going well and there is no pain. Others drop back care when work and family demands increase. If a lapse in your rehabilitation program has occurred, but a new back attack has not happened yet, quickly resume your exercises. Don't make yourself miserable with useless guilt, but do remember that recurrence of pain is likely unless rehabilitative measures are conscientiously and continuously pursued. Recovery is an ongoing process.

When you realize that it has been a few days (or a few weeks) since you have practiced your yoga, don't expect to resume exactly where you left off. You have probably lost some of what you gained during your previous work with the exercises. The best course of action is to return to the poses of Chapter 5, "Relaxation Techniques," and work there for a while. When you feel ready, move on to Chapter 6, "Home Base Poses." Work through this chapter at your own speed, adding new exercises and increasing the difficulty as you feel ready.

Avoid hurrying through the review. The key to safe back rehabilitation is working at the level appropriate for that moment. It is counterproductive to try to resume work at the level you had attained before your lapse.

Setbacks: What To Do If Pain Recurs

Sometimes a lapse lasts until a full-blown back attack occurs. Sometimes, too, you will have an attack even though you have been following your yoga regimen faithfully. It would be unrealistic to expect that once you have begun the program outlined in this book, you will never experience back pain again. Use this knowledge in a positive way. Look forward to using whatever setbacks occur for further refinement of your practice of

3.1

Back Care Diary

Date	Circumstances/Causes of Back Attack	Pain Duration	Location & Severity (Mild/Moderate/Extreme)	Comments
1.7.91	Lifted flower pot	3 days	lower back/ moderate	next time — get help!
5.5.91	Family stress; no exercise for 3. mos.	3 days	upper back/ neck	will do 5-10 minutes of my exercises first thing in the morning

3.1   Back Care Diary, Sample Entry

rehabilitative yoga. When a setback occurs, don't be surprised or discouraged. Use your recovery from each setback to help you learn to avoid future ones.

Look closely at what happened prior to the back attack. What factors (physical and emotional) led to this recurrence of pain? Was there increased stress at work or at home? Had you slacked off of your yoga program? Were you too aggressive with your exercises? Had you added a new physical activity or exercise program? How did your signal spot feel just before the setback or during the early stages of the setback? Was there an accident or a reinjury? (If so, medical reassessment might be indicated.) Note the answers to these questions in your Back Care Diary. (See Appendix as well as sample entry, Figure 3.1.)

The answers to these questions can give you insight into how to modify your behavior, exercise, and stress management in order to avoid future setbacks.

A setback is also a time for reflection on how the current situation differs from previous ones. Did you catch the signs of an oncoming back attack earlier than you had previously? Is your stay in bed briefer than in the past? Had your pain-free interval been longer than the previous one? Do you feel that you know more about what to do this time? If the answer to any of these questions is *yes*, take heart! Your control over the situations affecting your back is increasing and your spinal health is improving. If the answer to one or more of these questions is *no*, don't give up. You will probably answer *yes* to these questions in the future if you continue with this rehabilitation program.

When a setback occurs, don't just stop exercising. During the time of acute pain, return to the exercises in Chapter 5, "Relaxation Techniques," that work best for you. Review Chapter 12, "The Yoga of Daily Living," and Chapter 13, "Exercising Safely." Then, as you feel ready, go back to Chapter 6, "Home Base Poses." Slowly work through the early stages with an increased level of awareness of your signal spot. Pay particular attention to those areas that need improvement, based on your assessment of what led to this most recent attack. Use the Back Care Diary to record each attack and its circumstances. (See Appendix.) This information will help you recognize negative and positive trends.

Additional Therapeutic Modalities

In the types of problems discussed in this book, rehabilitative yoga, improved biomechanics in daily activities, and constructive rest are the most important elements leading to prolonged recovery. However, some additional therapeutic modalities can be helpful. The pros and cons of each are discussed in the following text. They have a common limitation: They may give symptomatic relief, but they will not change your postural habits or teach you to cope with stress. Remember that using pain-relieving medication of any type can be counterproductive, because it decreases or eliminates the information your body is trying to send you about how your posture and movements are affecting your back and

and neck. If your pain is removed artificially, you will not have the natural biofeedback you need to make corrections.

Transcutaneous electrical nerve stimulation (TENS). With transcutaneous electrical nerve stimulation, electrical current is sent into the muscles through electrodes taped on the skin and connected to a small power source that can be worn on a belt. The current blocks the transmission of pain to the brain, helping to break the cycle in which muscle spasm produces pain that, in turn, produces more muscle spasm. This device can be helpful during an acute back attack, when muscles are in painful spasm. It can be rented through a surgical supply house or from your physical therapist. Having to apply the electrodes and wear the device is somewhat inconvenient, but this inconvenience may be worth it if some measure of pain relief is provided.

Warm packs and ice packs. Application of either heat or ice can be helpful with some back problems. Some people find relief from heat; others prefer ice. To apply ice, freeze a neatly folded wet towel in a leakproof plastic bag and lie on it in a position of constructive rest (see Chapter 5, "Relaxation Techniques"). Ice should be applied for only twenty minutes per hour. If heat works best for you, be sure to use a heating pad that has an automatic shutoff to help avoid burns should you fall asleep.

Steroidal anti-inflammatory medication. Steroids, which have powerful anti-inflammatory action, can be taken orally for a limited period of time or injected directly into an area of painful swelling. (The steroids used for back pain are not the same as the anabolic steroids used illegally by athletes to build muscle mass.) Because of cumulative detrimental effects to the body's immune system and tissues, steroids are not a long-term answer to back problems. They can, however, provide short-term relief and frequently help your doctor establish a diagnosis: If you receive significant relief using steroids, this indicates that some or all of the pain may be due to tissue swelling and inflammation in the affected area. Therefore, rehabilitative exercise and constructive relaxation will probably be effective.

Nonsteroidal anti-inflammatory drugs (NSAIDs). Nonsteroidal anti-inflammatory drugs are a class of drugs related to aspirin that reduce inflammation. Like aspirin, they may cause stomach irritation. As with steroids, the NSAIDs can provide symptomatic relief only if some of the pain is related to tissue swelling and inflammation. Also like steroids, a good response to the NSAIDs indicates that therapeutic exercise and constructive relaxation have a good chance of relieving the underlying cause of the pain.

Muscle relaxant drugs. Muscle relaxant drugs may provide short-term relief if pain is partially due to muscle spasm. Unfortunately, they do not work well for many people. The drugs that work best as muscle relaxants are tranquilizers. However, you must weigh the potentially addictive aspects of these drugs against the temporary symptomatic relief from the pain. The tranquilizer-type muscle relaxants also create an overlay of psychological effects that are not always positive. They can leave your mind in a fog, hindering your motivation to follow an exercise program and interfering with constructive stress management and good interpersonal relationships.

Corsets and braces. Corsets and braces can provide external support for the back, but are only helpful short term. With long-term use the back muscles weaken, leaving the spine even more vulnerable. However, braces may be necessary for those with severe osteoporosis, vertebral fractures, or postoperative back instability.

Massage. Although massage cannot be considered a back rehabilitation technique, it can provide some benefits. It can temporarily relieve painful muscle spasm and help you relax. A massage therapist can provide you with useful information about which muscles are tight and which are not, so you can focus on the tight areas with stretching exercises. Most important, massage allows you to experience the feeling of soft, relaxed muscles. For many people, this will be the first time in years that they have felt such muscle relaxation. Such an experience, combined with the realization that this is how their muscles should feel most of the time, can be quite instructive. Just knowing that such a state exists can help you return to it in deep relaxation practice.

Chiropractic manipulation. Many people with back challenges have found temporary relief from chiropractic adjustments. Chiropractors are well trained to assess posture and alignment. Chiropractors familiar with Iyengar-style yoga frequently refer their patients to yoga teachers, who can help the patients make long-term postural corrections that help them hold chiropractic adjustments longer. To see how this works, explore the feelings of postural change after a successful chiropractic adjustment. Try to maintain the feeling of relief by allowing your posture and movement to change in response to the adjustment. Simply returning to your old habits of posture and movement will result in a return of the old problems.

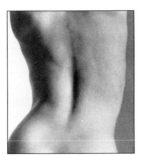

Four

Assessing Your Flexibility and Alignment

Is your back the real source of your pain, or is your back pain simply a symptom of a problem elsewhere in your body? For most people, the back is the victim of stresses and strains caused by misalignments in other areas. An apparent back problem may really be primarily a foot, knee, leg, hip, shoulder, or neck problem.

This chapter will help you evaluate alignment and flexibility throughout your body, so you can track down the source of your back pain. It will also show you which poses, or chapters in this book, to emphasize as you follow your yoga-based exercise and relaxation program. Even if you think you already know what is causing your back pain, do this assessment anyway—you may be surprised at the results. You may have a definite idea about what your strength, flexibility, and alignment are, based on old information or a body image left over from an earlier period in your life. However, it is likely that your alignment and flexibility have changed significantly over the years.

Give yourself permission to improve. This assessment reflects where you are now, not where you were ten or twenty years ago or where you will be after conscientious work. Your body is not poured in concrete. All of the tissues (even bones and scars) are malleable and can be realigned with persistent, intelligent effort. Do not accept your current alignment and flexiblity as a condemnation, but rather understand that where you are now is a starting point against which your future improvements can be measured. Each time you accept your current limitations and misalignments by saying, "This is how I am," you give yourself permission not to change. Instead, tell yourself, "My back is improving" or "This exercise is helping realign my spine." Your body hears and believes what you say. Be sure to give yourself encouragement and permission to improve at every opportunity.

Flexibility and Back Pain

Remember that it is not enough just to be flexible. Although back pain most often affects inflexible people, problems also occur for those with normal as well as greater than normal flexibility.

Normal flexibility will not prevent back pain if you have poor posture, poor body mechanics, an inactive lifestyle, or recent or remote trauma. Greater than normal flexibility, also known as *ligamentous laxity,* can actually predispose a person to back and joint injury when the muscles are not strong enough to provide stability and support for the joints. Ligaments become overstretched and joints deteriorate from the resultant excessive movement.

Fortunately for all—the inflexible, the normally flexible, and the overly flexible —this yoga-based exercise program provides whatever is needed. The inflexible become more flexible while learning improved posture and body mechanics. The overly flexible develop the muscular strength necessary to hold their joints in good alignment. And everyone develops better habits of posture, better habits of movement, and better balance among the interacting muscle groups.

Alignment and Flexibility Self-Assessment

As you go through the following tests of flexibility and alignment, use the Flexibility and Alignment Worksheet in the Appendix to keep track of your posture and flexibility. (See sample Flexibility and Alignment Worksheet entry at the end of this chapter, Figure 4.36.) Compare your right side with your left side. Following each test are suggestions for specific yoga postures that will improve strength and flexibility in the part of the body being tested. If you are weak in a particular area, emphasize these suggested postures as you practice your yoga routines. Document your progress by repeating these tests every three to six months and recording the results on your worksheet. "Notes" at the end of each test provide tips for those with special conditions.

Have a friend take photos of you performing the different alignment tests so you can clearly see where you are. The photos will give you precise information about your current posture and alignment for future comparison. Be sure to date them.

These tests are designed to be safe and painless. If one of them causes discomfort, reread the directions and repeat the test, stretching less intensely. If discomfort persists, note it on your worksheet. If you continue to have problems in this part of your body as you progress through the exercises, you may wish to consult an Iyengar-style yoga teacher (see Resources) or another health care professional.

Remember that no one is entirely symmetrical. You may have minor, insignificant misalignments. But if you have slight misalignments in a problem area or an area in which you have pain or other symptoms, pay attention to them and work on correcting them.

Use the information you gain through these tests as you practice the exercises later in the book. Understanding your asymmetries and misalignments is the first step toward correcting them.

Evaluation of Lumbar Curve

Because a simple visual assessment can be deceptive, the best way to evaluate your lumbar curve is with a hands-on approach. The following two personal anatomy lessons will help you evaluate your own lumbar curve.

Seated evaluation. You'll need a firm chair with a flat seat. If possible, place the chair next to a long mirror so that you can see yourself from the side. If you don't have a mirror, you can still perform this examination, using the tactile feedback from your hands.

Sit on your sitting bones (not your tailbone or sacrum) on the forward half of the chair seat. Place one hand on your lumbar spine (at the back of your waist). Place the other hand on the side waist at the top of the pelvis (Figure 4.1).

Now arch your back and tilt your pelvis forward so your navel moves forward toward your knees. Feel how this action increases your lumbar curve to a more swaybacked position. Feel how your pelvis has tilted forward (Figure 4.2).

Now move your navel toward your spine and tuck your tailbone. With the hand on the top of the pelvis, feel how the pelvis tilts backward (Figure 4.3). With the hand at the back waist, feel how the lumbar spine flattens. Notice that when your lumbar spine is flattened, the normal groove down the center of your back disappears, and you feel instead the bony ends of the spinous processes, the projections at the back of the vertebrae.

Perform these actions several times, so you understand the range of positions of the lumbar spine, from increased arch (swayback), through normal curve, to decreased arch (flat back).

Now sit in your usual posture and assess how your usual lumbar curve compares to these positions.

Standing evaluation. Stand with one side to a mirror. Bend your knees slightly to allow your pelvis to move freely. Place your hands as before, with one at the side waist on top of the pelvis, the other behind the waist on your lumbar spine (Figure 4.4).

Observing yourself from the side, again tip your pelvis forward, so that the lumbar curve is increased to a more swaybacked position (Figure 4.5). Feel how this motion changes the lumbar spine beneath your hand.

Now tilt your pelvis backward by squeezing the buttocks together and tightening the abdominal muscles, while tucking the tailbone and moving the pubic bone up toward the breastbone. Feel how your lower back flattens, and notice that your head simultaneously moves forward, your chest collapses, and your upper back rounds (Figure 4.6).

This evaluation gives you a good understanding of how your own lumbar spine can move through its range of motion from extension (forward tilt of the pelvis with an increased lumbar curve) to flexion (backward tilt of the pelvis with a flattened lumbar spine). Now straighten your knees and stand in your usual posture. Observe the position of your lumbar spine and compare it to the range of positions you have just explored. Is your lumbar spinal curve increased, normal, or flattened?

The effect of your lumbar curve upon the well-being of your back is enormous. In swayback, as you have just seen, the arch in the lower back is abnormally increased—typically, the belly protrudes in front, and the buttocks stick out behind. The ligaments that should support the spine become slack, and the weight that should have been evenly distributed over the entire lumbar curve becomes concentrated at the peak or point of the arch. This potent combination—instability plus an abnormal concentration of pressure at the center of the lumbar arch—allows excessive movement between vertebrae and contributes to disc deterioration and reactive bone changes, such as bone spurs (in which the bone actually grows in an abnormal way in an attempt to make itself strong enough to bear the stresses placed upon it).

By pinching together the back portions of the vertebrae, swayback creates chronic compression on the back of the lumbar discs, the pads that separate the vertebrae. This prolonged compression interrupts the flow of nourishment, and the discs begin to deteriorate and shrink. As the disc shrinks, the surfaces of the facet joints (the joints between the bony processes of the vertebrae) are no longer held apart at the proper distance, and they begin to grate against each other, eventually causing a type of arthritis. Abnormally functioning facet joints place additional stresses on the disc; thus, a vicious cycle of injury and deterioration is established.

With a flat back, the normal lumbar arch is flattened or greatly decreased and the buttocks appear to be tucked under. This posture often occurs in back patients who have overcorrected an increased lumbar curve. For many years back patients were given only flexion exercises, in which the lumbar curve was flattened. Repeated practice of these exercises and misguided efforts at walking and moving with a flat lumbar curve frequently created a new back problem.

Like swayback, the flat lumbar curve can create serious problems. Loss of the normal curve interferes with the spine's shock absorption. Flattening the curve makes the supporting ligaments taut, causing the vertebrae to be held tightly together. This limits motion and compromises disc nourishment. It also forces onto the discs the weight usually borne by the facet joints, resulting in compression, poor disc nourishment, and disc degeneration.

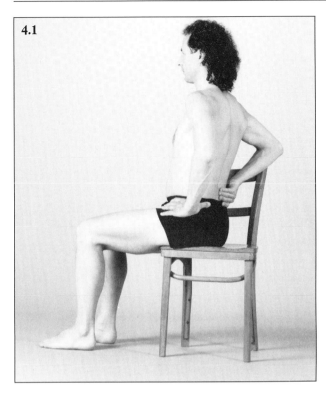

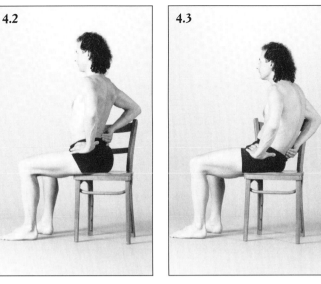

4.1   Seated Evaluation of Lumbar Curve, Normal
4.2   Seated Evaluation of Lumbar Curve, Swayback
4.3   Seated Evaluation of Lumbar Curve, Flat Back

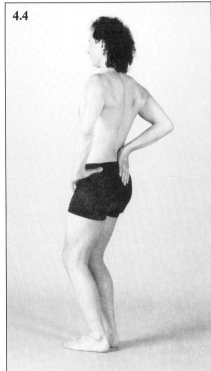

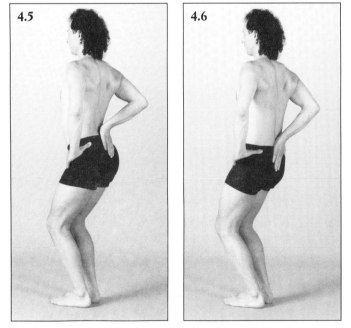

4.4   Standing Evaluation of Lumbar Curve, Normal
4.5   Standing Evaluation of Lumbar Curve, Swayback
4.6   Standing Evaluation of Lumbar Curve, Flat Back

Notes

- *If you have a swayback or a flat back, diligently practice all of the poses in Chapter 5, "Relaxation Techniques"; Chapter 6, "Home Base Poses"; and Chapter 7, "Moving On Poses."*
- *If you have a flat back, be sure to use a lumbar pad (Figure 5.6) when the poses call for lying on your back.*

Evaluation of Thoracic Curve

If you try to evaluate your thoracic (upper back) curve from the side without actually looking at your spine in the mirror, you can be fooled into thinking your back is rounded if your shoulder blades are prominent. Here's a way to evaluate your thoracic curve accurately.

Stand with your back at an angle to a mirror so you can look over your shoulder and see your upper spine. If you can reach, place one hand on your upper spine, with your fingers touching the center of your back just below your neck. If you can't reach, just observe your spine in the mirror. Stand as straight as you can and feel the skin of your upper back between your shoulder blades. If your alignment is correct, the skin should feel smooth, with no protruding vertebrae, as you slide your fingers from one shoulder blade to the other (Figure 4.7).

Now slump forward and round your upper back as much as possible. When you do this, you will feel the vertebrae protrude into a lump along the midline (Figure 4.8). Look in the mirror and view your upper spine's range of motion, from your best erect posture to the slumped position. (Also notice if your spine is so stiff that you cannot perceive a difference in the two positions.) Now stand as you normally would and see if your upper back is rounded or erect.

Note

- *If your upper back is excessively rounded, practice the poses in Chapter 9, "Rounded Upper Back, Forward Head Posture, and Neck Pain."*

Evaluation of Shoulder Roundedness and Shoulder Blade Position

Stand facing a mirror and observe your shoulders. Roll your shoulders forward and back (Figures 4.9A and 4.9B). As you roll your shoulders forward, you will notice a hollow indentation where each shoulder joins your chest. This hollow indicates that the shoulders are in an abnormal and vulnerable position. As you roll your shoulders back, this indentation will disappear.

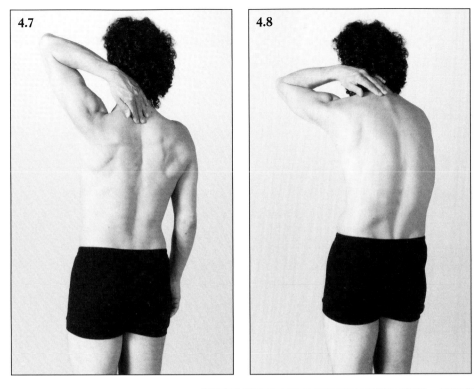

4.7   Evaluation of Thoracic
        Curve, Normal
4.8   Evaluation of Thoracic
        Curve, Rounded Upper
        Back
4.9A Evaluation of Shoulders,
        Normal
4.9B Evaluation of Shoulders,
        Rounded

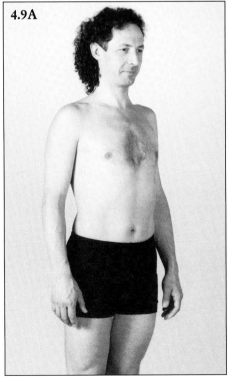

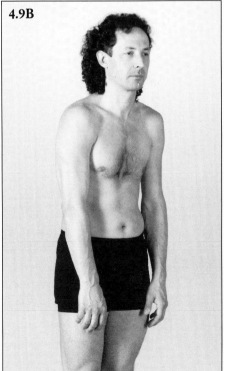

Now stand with your back to the mirror so you can look over your shoulder and observe your shoulder blades. Roll the shoulders forward so that the hollows are created on the front of the chest. In the mirror, notice that your shoulder blades slide upward and protrude further (Figure 4.10). Now roll the shoulders back so the indentations on the front of the chest disappear. At the same time, notice that the shoulder blades are moving downward and becoming flatter (Figure 4.11). This latter position is the healthy one for proper shoulder alignment. This shoulder position encourages the proper relationship of the upper back to the neck.

Now stand in your normal posture. What position do your shoulder blades naturally assume?

Note

• *If your shoulders are rounded, emphasize Wall Push (Figure 7.25), as well as all the poses in Chapter 9, "Rounded Upper Back, Forward Head Posture, and Neck Pain."*

Evaluation of Standing Alignment

Ask a friend to help check your alignment against a plumb line. Tie a small weight to one end of a string and attach the other end to the ceiling or a doorway. To evaluate your alignment from the side, stand so that the string is one inch in front of the center of the outside anklebone. To evaluate alignment from the back, stand so the string falls midway between the heels.

Viewed from the side, a line just in front of the ankle should pass upward through the centers of the knee joint, hip joint, and shoulder to the ear hole (Figure 4.12). This alignment places the heavy structures of the head, chest, and abdomen over the weight-bearing portions of your spine and legs. If your head or shoulders are forward of the line, you have *forward head position*. This posture may be accompanied by an increase in the thoracic (upper back) curve. (If you have forward head position or a rounded upper back, see Chapter 9.). If the center of your knee joint is behind the line, you may have *hyperextended* (overstraightened) knees. If your knees are partly bent, they will be in front of the line.

When you stand in front of the plumb bob, the line should pass through the center of the back of your head, the center of each vertebra, the cleft of the buttocks, midway between the knees, and midway between the heels (Figure 4.13). Minor variations are frequent and usually not clinically significant. If an area of misalignment is painful, however, then it is probably significant and may be related to scoliosis (Figure 4.14).

Note

• *If your knees are hyperextended, practice Mountain Pose (Figure 6.22).*

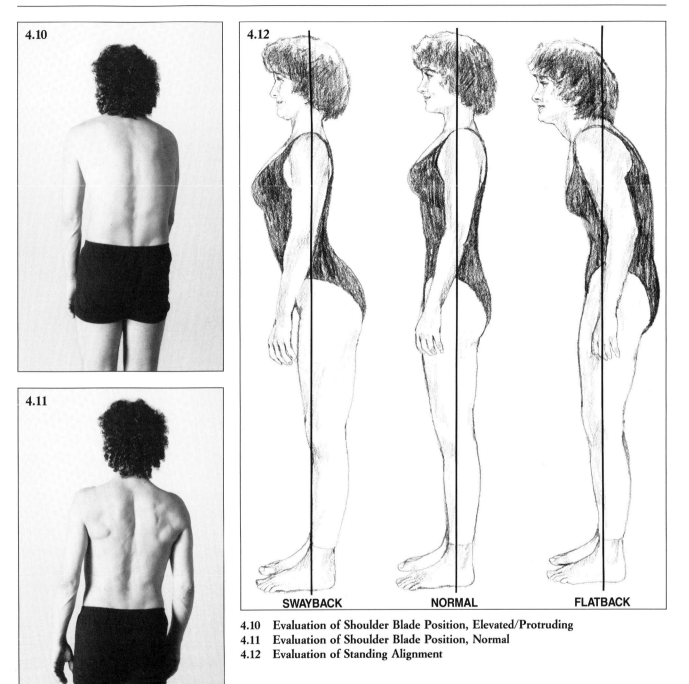

SWAYBACK   NORMAL   FLATBACK

4.10   Evaluation of Shoulder Blade Position, Elevated/Protruding
4.11   Evaluation of Shoulder Blade Position, Normal
4.12   Evaluation of Standing Alignment

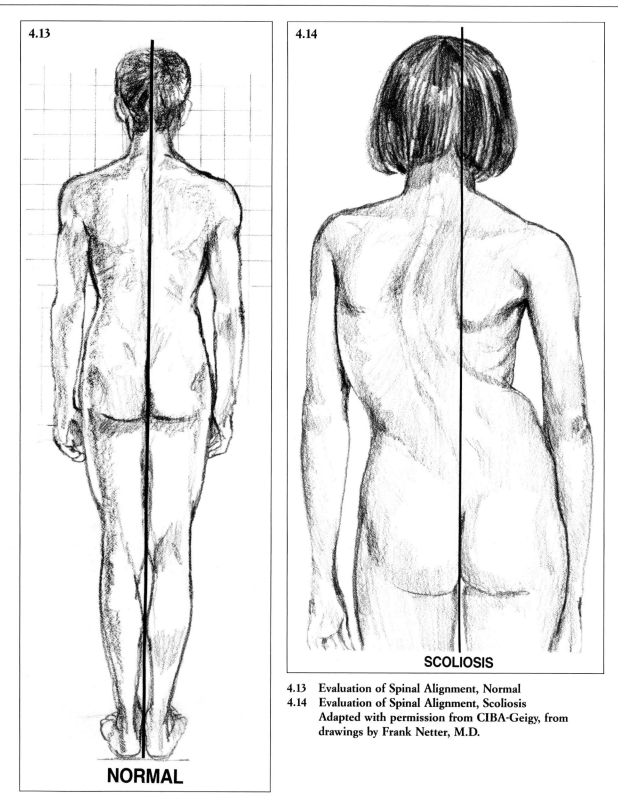

4.13

NORMAL

4.14

SCOLIOSIS

4.13   Evaluation of Spinal Alignment, Normal
4.14   Evaluation of Spinal Alignment, Scoliosis
Adapted with permission from CIBA-Geigy, from
drawings by Frank Netter, M.D.

Evaluation for Possible Scoliosis

Examine your ribs before a mirror. Are the ribs on one side more prominent? Is one shoulder higher than the other? These differences may reflect scoliosis (side-to-side spinal curvature).

To determine whether you have scoliosis, sit on a firm chair with an observer standing behind you. Bend forward at the hips while your observer evaluates your back for symmetry. With true scoliosis (a curvature that is part of the structure of the spine), one side of the back rib cage will be more prominent than the other (Figure 4.15).

With functional scoliosis (curvature which is not inherent in the structure of the spine, but is caused by other variables, such as imbalances in the pelvis) any curvature which exists while standing up will not be apparent in this forward bending test.

Note

• *If you have scoliosis, emphasize the poses in Chapter 10, "Scoliosis," in addition to the Relaxation, Home Base, and Moving On poses.*

Evaluation for Level Pelvis

Stand in front of a mirror and stretch a tape from the front of one hipbone at its highest point to the other. The tape should run exactly parallel to the floor (Figure 4.16).

If the tape is at an angle, this could indicate a short leg, scoliosis, asymmetry in the length of the muscles that support and balance the pelvis, or asymmetry in the pelvic bones. One leg may appear shorter than the other if one leg is weak, one foot is pronated (collapsed inward), or one knee hyperextends or collapses inward. There can also be an actual difference in the lengths of the leg bones.

Note

• *If your pelvis is not level, be sure to carefully evaluate your knee, ankle, and foot alignment, as these can contribute to pelvic distortion. Also pay special attention to the Evaluation for Sacroiliac Joint Asymmetry (Figures 4.26–4.28), as this condition is often present when the pelvis is not level. Emphasize Mountain Pose (Figure 6.22) and all the poses in Chapter 7, "Moving On Poses."*

Evaluation of the Knees

Stand with your feet parallel in front of a mirror and bend your knees. Do your knees come together in the midline (Figure 4.17), splay apart, or move straight out over your toes (Figure 4.18)? Straighten your knees fully (Figure 4.19). Do they separate widely as you straighten them (Figure 4.20)?

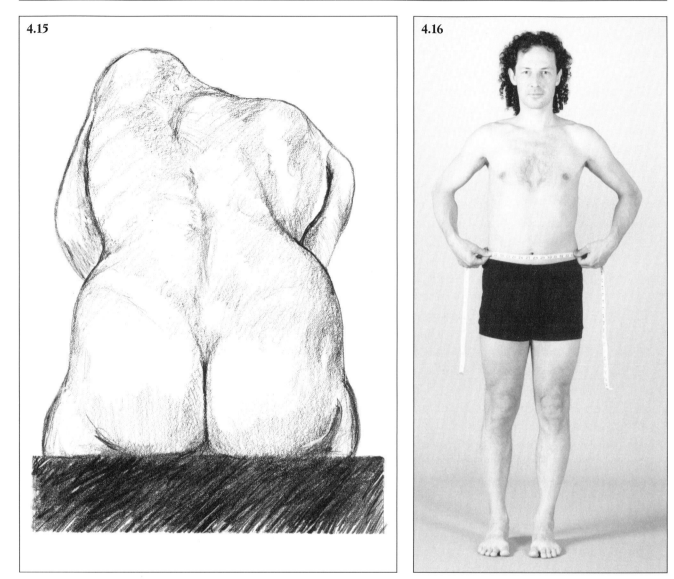

4.15 True Scoliosis, Prominent Ribs on One Side
Adapted with permission from CIBA-Geigy, from drawings by
Frank Netter, M.D.
4.16 Tape Measure Test for Level Pelvis

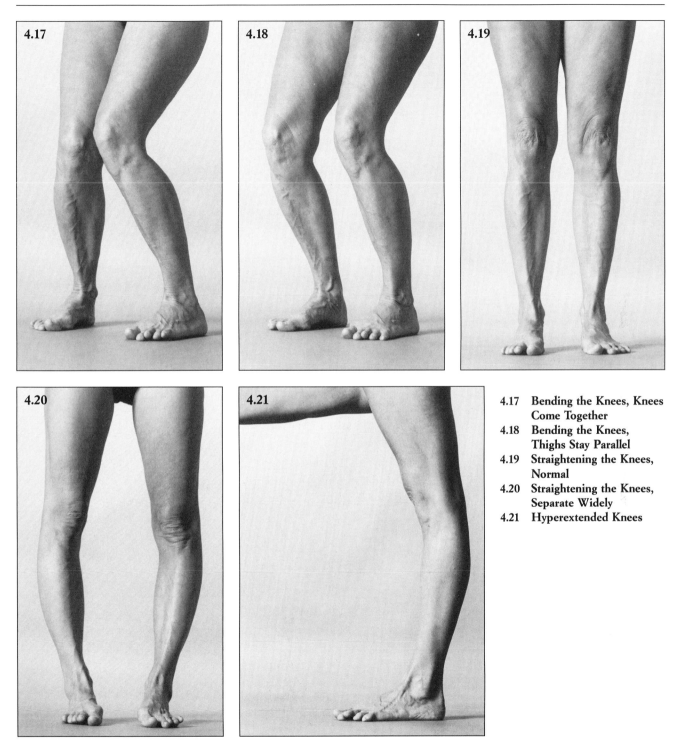

4.17 Bending the Knees, Knees Come Together
4.18 Bending the Knees, Thighs Stay Parallel
4.19 Straightening the Knees, Normal
4.20 Straightening the Knees, Separate Widely
4.21 Hyperextended Knees

If your knees come together or separate widely as you bend and straighten them, there is an imbalance in the muscles controlling the bending and straightening of the knees. When you straighten your knees, if they move toward each other when they are aligned over your ankles and then separate widely as they straighten even more, you may have *hyperextended* (overstraightened) knees (Figure 4.21). This condition causes a bow-legged appearance but is not a true bone deformity.

Knee misalignments, frequently associated with flat feet and swayback, can cause excessive pressure on the front part of the pelvis at the hip joint. The abnormal forces on the knee joint can cause it to deteriorate.

Note

• *If you have knee misalignments, emphasize Mountain Pose (Figure 6.22). Also work diligently with all of the Moving On poses in Chapter 7.*

Evaluation of Ankle and Foot Alignment

Have someone stand behind you and evaluate the relationship of your heels and ankles. If the heels and ankles lean inward or outward, this misalignment creates abnormal forces on the feet, knees, and hips. Does one foot lean in or out more than the other? Are your arches flattened?

Do you have claw toes, hammer toes, bunions, or big toes that deviate away from the midline? Claw toes have the first and second joints fixed in a claw position. With hammer toes, the first joints (the ones closest to the foot) are fixed in a straight position, but the end joints can bend, giving the appearance of a hammer. Both claw toes and hammer toes can be aggravated by arthritis. These toe configurations usually result from poor weight distribution on the feet, which causes the toes to try to grip the floor for stability. Big toes that deviate away from the midline are usually caused by narrow, pointed-toe shoes and may lead to painful bunions. The resultant poor weight distribution has negative repercussions on the ankles, knees, and lower back.

Note

• *If your ankles and feet are misaligned, go barefoot as often as possible and always practice your yoga barefoot. Make sure your shoes have enough room for your toes to spread out just as if you were barefoot. Emphasize Mountain Pose (Figure 6.22). Also see Chapter 7 for foot tips for the standing poses.*

Evaluation of Shoulder Flexibility

Lie on your back with your knees bent and your feet flat on the floor. Place a folded towel behind your head for support. Press your lower back to the floor and keep it there. Stretch both arms overhead. Your hands should rest easily on the floor while your lower back remains flat on the floor (Figure 4.22).

If your hands do not reach the floor or if you can't keep your lower back on the floor, your ability to raise your arms is significantly limited (Figure 4.23). This limitation in shoulder flexibility can place excessive demands on the lower back when reaching overhead.

Note

- *If your shoulders are tight, emphasize Wall Push (Figure 7.25). In Chapter 9, practice Arm Raises (Figures 9.6, 9.7), Entwine the Forearms (Figure 9.10), and One Elbow Up, One Elbow Down (Figure 9.12).*

Evaluation of Hip Flexibility

Lie on your back with both knees bent and your lower back touching the floor. Hold one knee to your chest and stretch the other leg out on the floor (Figure 4.24). If the knee of the outstretched leg can't be fully straightened, this indicates tightness of the hip flexor muscles, which cross the hip joint in the front of the thigh (Figure 4.25). These muscles, which include the quadriceps and the iliopsoas, act to raise the thigh toward the chest. (See also Figures 2.7A, 2.7B.) One end of the iliopsoas attaches to the inner side of the pelvis and the spine, and the other end attaches to the upper inner thighbone. Therefore, a tight iliopsoas pulls on the spine, causing an abnormal, stressful increase in the lumbar curve. Tight quadriceps (the muscles of the front thigh) can also increase the lumbar curve, by pulling the pubic bone down toward the legs.

Note

- *If your hip flexors are tight, emphasize One Leg Up, One Leg Out (Figure 6.15), Kneeling Lunge (Figure 6.17), Standing Twist (Figure 6.25), and Easy Bridge Pose (Figures 6.12, 6.13) in Chapter 6, "Home Base Poses." In Chapter 7, "Moving On Poses," emphasize Triangle Pose (Figure 7.4), Half-Moon Pose (Figure 7.14), Warrior Pose (Figure 7.18), and One-Legged Wall Push (Figure 7.29).*

Evaluation of Sacroiliac Joint Asymmetry

If you place the heel of your hand below your waist and the tip of the middle finger on your tailbone, your palm will be over the flat triangular bone called the *sacrum* (Figure 4.26). The *sacroiliac (SI) joints* are the bony knobs on either side of the top of the sacrum, where it meets the wing-shaped bones of the pelvis. To feel your SI joints, hook your thumbs over your hips, thumbs pointing forward and fingertips pointing toward each other below your waist. The tips of your fingers will end up on the slight bulges marking the SI joints (Figure 4.27).

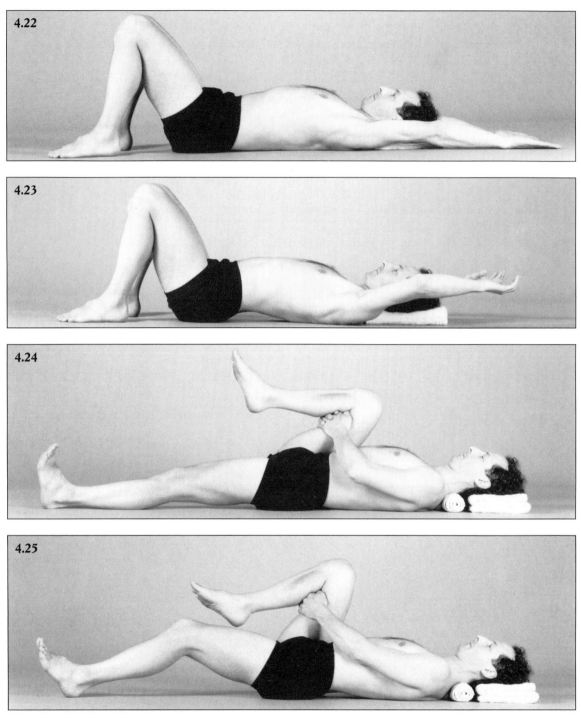

4.22 Shoulder Flexibility Test, Normal
4.23 Shoulder Flexibility Test, Limited
4.24 Hip Flexibility Test, Normal
4.25 Hip Flexibility Test, Decreased Flexibility

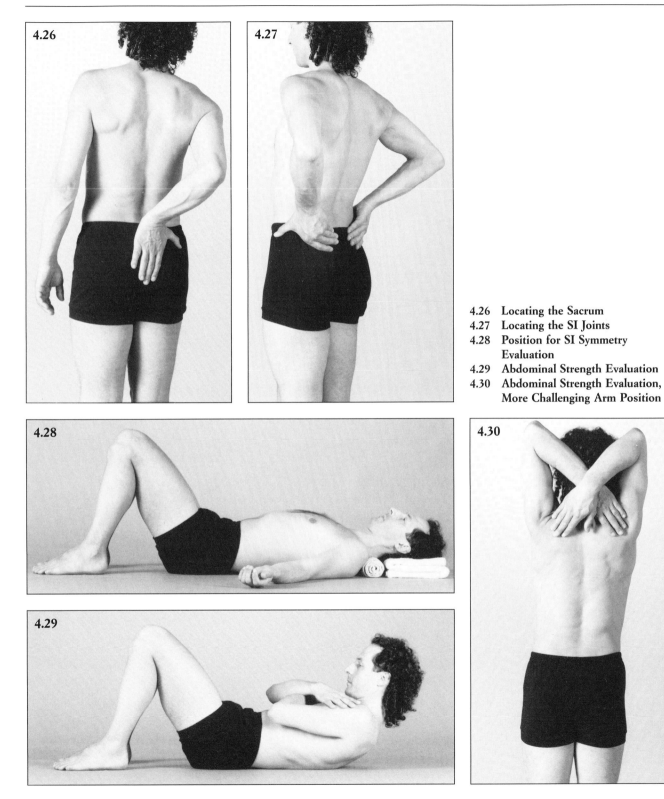

4.26   Locating the Sacrum
4.27   Locating the SI Joints
4.28   Position for SI Symmetry
        Evaluation
4.29   Abdominal Strength Evaluation
4.30   Abdominal Strength Evaluation,
        More Challenging Arm Position

Lie on your back with your knees bent and a folded towel behind your head. Keeping your knees together, move them from side to side so that you feel the pressure of your sacrum against the floor (Figure 4.28). Evaluate whether one SI joint feels sharper or more pointed and whether the other side feels caved in or depressed. Also note if one side is tender.

If you feel a difference between the two sides, you may have pelvic torsion, a twisting of the pelvis at the sacroiliac joint that causes compression of one SI joint and over-stretching of the other. This condition can be caused by scoliosis (abnormal side-to-side spinal curves), leg-length discrepancies, one hamstring muscle group much tighter than the other, trauma to the pelvis or spine, habitually sitting crosslegged, habitually standing with the weight on one leg, and playing such asymmetric sports as golf and tennis. Pelvic torsion places unequal stresses on the hips, knees, sacroiliac joints, and right and left sides of the spine.

Note

- *If your sacroiliac joints are asymmetrical, see Chapter 8, "Sacroiliac Pain and Sciatica."*

Evaluation of Abdominal Strength

If you have a forward head position or rounded upper back, you will need a folded towel or blanket for this test. Lie on your back with your knees bent and the folded towel or blanket behind your head. Cross your arms in front of your chest. Now raise your head and shoulders from the floor (Figure 4.29). *Do not lift all the way into a complete sitting position.*

If lifting your head and shoulders is easy, try it with a more challenging arm position. Cross your forearms behind your head, touching each shoulder with the opposite hand (Figure 4.30), or hold each earlobe with the thumb and finger of each hand. (*Do not hold the back of your head with your hands.*) Now lift your head and shoulders from the floor. If you can't do it, return to the first position and see how many head and shoulder lifts you can do. If you can lift your head and shoulders from the floor in the more difficult arm positions, see how many times you can do it.

You have very weak abdominal muscles if you are unable to lift your head and shoulders from the floor at all.

Your abdominal muscles are moderately weak if you are able to lift your head and shoulders from the floor, with your arms crossed in front of your chest, fewer than five times.

You have moderately strong abdominal muscles if you are able to lift your head and shoulders in either of the more challenging arms positions more than ten times.

Note

- *If your abdominal muscles need strengthening, emphasize Supine Pelvic Tilt (Figure 6.1), Yoga Sit-Ups (Figures 6.3, 6.4), and Supine Knee-Chest Twist, variation 2 (Figure 6.6).*

Evaluation of Hamstring Flexibility

Sit with one side next to a wall, knees bent and feet on the floor. Using your arms to support your body, lie down on your side with your buttocks close to the wall and your head away from it. Keeping your knees bent toward your chest, roll over onto your back. Place a folded towel behind your head for comfort. Gradually straighten your legs, sliding your heels up the wall (Figure 4.31).

If your knees can't be fully straightened or if your buttocks and sacrum aren't on the floor (Figure 4.32), move your buttocks away from the wall until your sacrum is firmly on the floor and your knees can straighten completely (Figure 4.33). Note the distance from your buttocks to the wall. If you have to move your buttocks more than two inches away from the wall in order to fully straighten your knees, you have a significant degree of tightness in the hamstrings, the long, powerful muscles at the back of the thigh.

Because the hamstrings attach to the sitting bones (the bony protuberances at the base of the pelvis), shortened hamstrings prevent normal movement of the pelvis and can flatten the lumbar curve. Tight hamstrings put the lower back at risk by preventing the pelvis from tilting when you bend forward, thus requiring all the movement to come from the lower back.

Note

- *If your hamstrings are tight, emphasize One Leg Up, One Leg Out (Figure 6.14, 6.15) and Standing Twist (Figure 6.24, 6.25) in Chapter 6, "Home Base Poses." All of the Moving On poses in Chapter 7 are also important.*

Evaluation of Inner Thigh Flexibility

Lie in the same position as for the hamstring flexibility test (buttocks and sacrum on the floor and the legs up the wall, knees straight, a folded towel behind your head). Start with both legs together, heels against the wall. Let your legs fall away from each other toward the floor so that they form a **V**. The angle of the legs should be about ninety degrees (Figure 4.34). (If there is pain in the inner side of your knee, pull your toes back toward your head as you stretch outward with the heel. If that doesn't work, bring your legs closer together.) On your worksheet, note the angle between the thighs and whether each foot is about the same distance from the floor. To come out of the position, use your hands to push your legs back together.

If the angle of your legs is less than ninety degrees, your inner thigh muscles (*adductors*) need to be stretched. If the inner thigh muscles are tight, they pull the pubic bone down, tilting the pelvis forward and increasing the lumbar curve. They can also pull the thighbone inward, creating knock-knees. In runners, tight adductors can cause instability and irritation in the pubic area by pulling the two sides of the pubic bone in opposite directions.

Note

- *If your inner thighs are tight, rest in the test position just described for thirty to sixty seconds per day. Practice One Leg Up, One Leg Out (Figures 6.14, 6.15). All of the Moving On poses in Chapter 7 will also be helpful.*

Overweight

If you are overweight, you don't need a test to tell you so. But you do need to understand how your weight may be affecting your back. Excess weight concentrated in the abdomen can alter lumbar mechanics and make your lower back vulnerable to injury. Excess fat in the tissues surrounding the intestines causes the contents of the abdomen to push out against the abdominal wall, stretching and lengthening the abdominal muscles, which decreases their ability to support the lumbar spine from the front. The change in your center of gravity, due to the accumulation of fat, increases pressures on the lumbar discs.

Excess weight increases the load on your knees and ankles and exacerbates any misalignments in your feet, ankles, or knees. This can lead to arthritis in the affected joints.

Note

- *If you are overweight, dealing successfully with overweight may require professional help through a structured program offering education in behavior modification, nutrition, and exercise. The body mechanics principles in Chapter 12, "The Yoga of Daily Living," are especially important for healthy reconstructive exercise.*

Injuries or Special Conditions

In addition to assessing your flexibility and alignment, it is important that you take into consideration any special spinal conditions or injuries you might have, such as spondylolysis, spondylolisthesis, spinal stenosis, and spinal arthritis. These conditions cannot be assessed through a simple test. But if you have already been diagnosed with these conditions, the following information will help you understand how they might affect your exercise program.

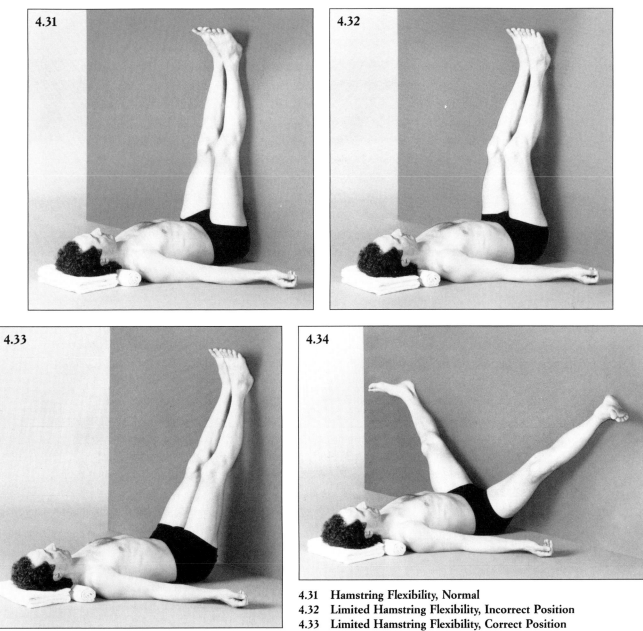

4.31   Hamstring Flexibility, Normal
4.32   Limited Hamstring Flexibility, Incorrect Position
4.33   Limited Hamstring Flexibility, Correct Position
4.34   Inner Thigh Flexibility, Normal

Spondylolysis and Spondylolisthesis

Spondylolysis and spondylolisthesis are two closely related disorders of the lumbar spine in which the connections between the vertebrae weaken and break. In spondylolysis, the vertebrae separate on just one side. This fracture allows the bones to move too much, grinding down the intervertebral discs.

In spondylolisthesis, the connections break on both sides of the vertebra, and the vertebral body slips forward over the next lower one (Figure 4.35). The disc at the slippage site rapidly degenerates. At first, the condition may be without symptoms. When symptoms do occur, they are related to nerve or spinal cord compression, which can produce leg, buttock, hip, or foot pain, or numbness or weakness on one or both sides.

Gymnasts, bowlers, and rowers often experience these conditions as a result of trauma, since these sports encourage the upper part of the body to slide forward over the lower part.

Notes

- *If you have spondylolysis or spondylolisthesis, practice the Home Base and Moving On poses in Chapters 6 and 7, observing the specific cautions given for people with these conditions. In general, observe several basic principles when exercising:*
  - *To prevent the upper vertebrae from slipping forward over the lower ones, do not hold the trunk forward of the pelvis. Do not allow the arch in the lower back to increase. Avoid high heels, forward bends, and such exercises as rowing, bowling, gymnastics, and cycling.*
  - *Do movements that encourage the upper vertebrae to move backward over the lower ones, such as lying on your back and hugging your knees to your chest.*
  - *Strengthen muscles that can provide support for the lower back area, including the paraspinals (the muscles on either side of the spine), hip rotators, abdominals, and the leg and buttock muscles.*
  - *Increase flexibility elsewhere to avoid excessive demands for motion in the lumbosacral area. Increase the flexibility of the shoulder girdle, arms, and hip joints. Increase rotational flexibility in the upper back.*

Arthritis of the Spine

The facet joints of the spine can develop both major types of arthritis, rheumatoid arthritis and osteoarthritis (degenerative arthritis).

In *rheumatoid arthritis,* the joint lining becomes inflamed due to abnormal functioning of the immune system. The immune cells erroneously destroy the joint lining as if it were a foreign invader, such as bacteria or a fungus. When this process occurs in the

4.35

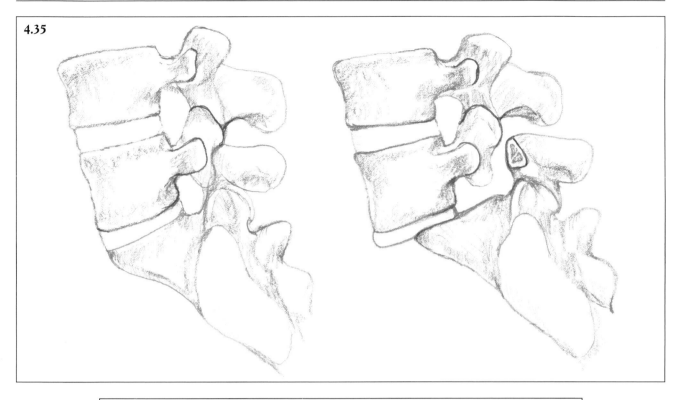

4.36

Flexibility and Alignment Worksheet

	Date ☞ 4.3.91	8.3.91	1.6.92
Seated Evaluation of Lumbar Curve (Figures 4.1–4.3) flat, normal, sway	sway	normal	normal
Standing Evaluation of Lumbar Curve (Figures 4.4–4.6) flat, normal, sway	sway	sway	normal
Evaluation of Thoracic Curve (Figures 4.7–4.8) increased, normal, decreased	decreased	decreased	normal
Evaluation of Right Shoulder Roundedness and Right Shoulder Blade Position (Figures 4.9–4.11) rounded, normal, high, low	rounded high	rounded high	normal
Evaluation of Left Shoulder Roundedness and Left Shoulder Blade Position (Figures 4.9–4.11) rounded, normal, high, low	rounded normal	rounded normal	normal
Evaluation of Standing Alignment from Side (Figure 4.12) Head forward, normal, back	forward	forward	normal

4.35   Spondylolisthesis. Adapted with permission from *The Intervertebral Disc* by A.F.
       dePalma and R.H. Rothman. Philadelphia: W.B. Saunders Co., 1970.
4.36   Flexibility and Alignment Worksheet, Sample Entry

joints of the spine (a condition referred to as *ankylosing spondylitis),* the inflammation of the spine's facet joints causes the vertebrae to become fused together, so the spine becomes rigid and inflexible. (This condition's X-ray resemblance to a stalk of bamboo is responsible for its more well known name, *bamboo spine.*) The pain and immobility result in muscle weakness. The unstimulated vertebrae lose calcium and become fragile and porous because of the decrease in weight-bearing activity and exercise.

Osteoarthritis (also known as degenerative arthritis or degenerative joint disease) is commonly thought to arise from the normal wear and tear on the joints that comes with age. In my experience, it is also frequently associated with long-standing incorrect body mechanics due to poor posture or alignment.

Osteoarthritis of the facet joints can result from chronic postural strain (for example, flat back, swayback, scoliosis, forward head, or any other postural or mechanical problems) that causes abnormal forces on the joints. The gliding surfaces of these joints become roughened and irregular, and the lining of the joint becomes scarred. In an attempt to buttress the facets to enhance weight bearing in these abnormal situations, the bones may produce spurs, which sometimes impinge upon joints, nerves, and soft tissues, limiting movement or creating pain.

A diagnosis of spinal arthritis does not mean that nothing can be done about the resultant back pain. The exercises in this book will help improve posture and decrease the abnormal demands on the spinal joints. Because bone is a living, self-healing tissue, with time there may even be a reduction in the bony spurs, as posture and body mechanics improve. Don't take a diagnosis of arthritis to mean that the damage is irreparable. Take it as a signal to improve posture and body mechanics.

Note

- *If you have arthritis of the spine, approach exercise cautiously. Work under the close supervision of a physical or occupational therapist until your exercise tolerance is well delineated and you understand the principles of correct movement. Working with a yoga teacher experienced in therapeutic yoga, in conjunction with a physical therapist and a rheumatologist, can be a great team approach to rehabilitation.*
- *Start your yoga regimen with the Relaxation poses in Chapter 5. One at a time, gradually work your way through the Home Base poses in Chapter 6.*
- *If you also have a rounded upper back, add some poses from Chapter 9.*
- *As you feel ready, try the Moving On poses in Chapter 7.*

Lumbosacral Fusion and Other Congenital
Anomalies of the Lower Back

Several congenital defects in the bones of the lower lumbar vertebrae and sacrum are associated with back pain, including *sacralization of the fifth lumbar vertebra, lumbarization of the first sacral vertebra, asymmetry of lumbar facet joints,* and *spina bifida occulta.*

The normal sacrum is a large triangular bone formed by the fusion of the last five vertebrae. In sacralization of the fifth lumbar vertebra, one side of the last lumbar vertebra is fused into a single bone with the sacrum. A similar condition, lumbarization of the first sacral vertebra, occurs when the first sacral vertebra does not fuse into a single bone with the remainder of the sacral vertebrae. Instead, half of it is fused with the sacrum, while the other half has a structure more like that of a lumbar vertebra. In both of these conditions, the partially fused area is insufficiently mobile, creating compensatory hypermobility above it. The disc in the hypermobile segment degenerates and the joints subjected to increased movement can develop wear-and-tear arthritis.

In *spina bifida occulta,* the neural arches that form the spinal canal don't completely meet. This condition usually has no symptoms. People with spina bifida occulta who have back pain often blame their pain on their spina bifida, when in fact it is usually due to the same postural flaws and poor body mechanics that cause other people pain.

Another congenital anomaly of the lumbar spine involves asymmetry of the facet joints. Normal lumbar facet joints are designed to limit the rotation of the vertebra. If a facet joint surface is angled improperly, the joint moves much more freely. This can cause increased wear and tear on the neighboring discs.

Yoga therapy for such congenital defects aims to increase the strength of the muscles that can provide support for these abnormal structures (buttock, thigh, abdominal, and paraspinal muscles) and to decrease the excessive demands for movement and rotational strain at these areas by improving flexibility in the midback, shoulders, and hips.

Note

• *If you have any congenital anomalies of the lower back, follow a basic yoga regimen, including Relaxation poses (Chapter 5), Home Base poses (Chapter 6), and Moving On poses (Chapter 7). Pay attention to the yoga of daily living (Chapter 12).*

Spinal Stenosis and Old Spinal Fractures

Spinal stenosis is a condition in which bony overgrowth narrows the spinal canal, often impinging on the spinal cord. Sometimes congenital, this condition can also be related to previous spinal surgery, severe arthritis of the spine, or spondylolisthesis. Correction usually requires surgical removal of the excess bone.

Old fractures of the spine often result in scarring, which can render certain areas of the spine almost immobile. Other areas, in compensation, become hypermobile, resulting in disc degeneration and traumatic arthritis of the facet joints. Scar tissue from old fractures can also compress and irritate entrapped nerves.

Yoga rehabilitation in these two conditions is basically the same as with lumbosacral fusion and congenital anomalies of the lower back. The supporting muscles (buttock, thigh, abdominal, and paraspinal muscles) must be strengthened. At the same time, flexibility in the midback, shoulders, and hips must be improved, to decrease demands for movement and rotation in the lower back. Because of the unpredictability of the bone structure, it is difficult to predict whether the exercises for flatback or swayback will be more effective. Try both and use those which work the best for you.

Note

- *If you have spinal stenosis or old spinal fractures, follow a basic yoga regimen, including Relaxation poses (Chapter 5), Home Base poses (Chapter 6), and Moving On poses (Chapter 7). Pay attention to the yoga of daily living (Chapter 12).*

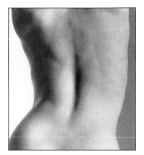

Five

Relaxation Techniques

A working mother's back goes out during preparations for her daughter's wedding.

- A businessman's back goes out just as he gets off the plane for his long-overdue vacation.
- Back pain erupts for a middle-aged woman in the midst of holiday preparations.
- Neck pain and tension headaches develop in the only family member capable of caring for an elderly parent.
- A young mother happily pregnant with her second baby finds that her back hurts so badly that she can no longer pick up her toddler.

Joy, responsibility, and tragedy can be stressful. This stress may lead to back pain. Many people who have recurrent back problems have observed that their back attacks seem to occur at "exactly the wrong time." Of course, there is never a good time to develop back pain, but it does seem to have a propensity for occurring when it is particularly inconvenient.

Yoga stretches and relaxation techniques can be powerful tools for coping with stress. While yoga can't make a stressful situation go away, it can change the way you perceive and respond to it.

The Effects of Stress

Being in danger or feeling helpless causes a specific set of physiological responses designed to prepare you to fight or flee. The fight or flight response is characterized by increases in heart rate, blood pressure, mental alertness, and muscle tension. This physiological response is appropriate in a life-threatening situation. But if it is maintained inappropriately, your quality of life—and even your life itself—can be threatened. A chronically stressed state can keep your body's healing mechanisms from working, prolonging recovery from injury or disease and leading to stress-related diseases, including ulcers, alcoholism, high blood pressure, depression, and, of course, back pain.

If you feel helpless, stress exaggerates your feelings of defeat and can lead to depression. Depression is accompanied by inactivity and the rounded shoulders, slumped spine, and hanging head of hopelessness. This combination of inactivity, a sense of defeat, and the body language of despair are powerful negative signals to give up the fight, which can lead to further deterioration in muscle strength, depression of your immune function, and the lowering of your ability to fight infection.

Stressful situations can heighten your dependency on others, especially when the stressful situation is complicated by recurrent pain or reinjury. If you are just beginning to feel independent again, the stress-induced recurrence of pain can be a blow to your feelings of autonomy, adding another layer of depression and hopelessness.

On the physical level, stress also exaggerates postural strain by increasing muscle tension. This increase in muscle tension does not occur uniformly throughout the body. Muscles that are already irritated, tense, or injured are more vulnerable. Any musculoskeletal misalignment is exaggerated, increasing the likelihood of reinjury.

The increased tension of a muscle at risk can cause it to go over the edge into spasm, an abnormal, painful state of muscle contraction in which the muscle will not release or relax. A spasm squeezes the blood vessels to the muscle, cutting off its nourishment. This causes the muscle metabolism to go into an anaerobic (without oxygen) mode in which lactic acid is produced. Lactic acid is a chemical messenger to the brain, telling it that you are under stress. In other words, a stressed muscle sends additional signals of stress throughout the body, further increasing overall muscle tension.

Gentle yoga stretches help break this self-perpetuating stress cycle. The brain perceives muscle stretch as the opposite of muscle tension. Whereas a muscle in spasm sends signals of danger to the entire body, the biofeedback from yoga muscle stretches is a signal of safety and well-being (Figure 5.1).

Coping Skills To Help You Deal with Stress

Whether a challenging event or circumstance has a stressful effect depends on your coping skills. Your reaction to a stressful event is related to:

- Whether you perceive the situation as threatening or undesirable
- Whether you feel you have some control over the situation
- Whether you respond to the challenge in ways that interfere with your taking care of yourself

When faced with a stressful situation that you cannot control, it is important for you to know that there are other elements of your life that you *can* control. *Control what you can*—this helps break the stress cycle by counteracting the negative effects of feelings of helplessness and hopelessness. In times of stress, it is crucial that you take care of yourself. Only then can you deal with a demanding situation or help others.

Among the things that you can control are your posture and body language, muscular tension, breathing, exercise, and diet. Some of the ways of practicing control and of exhibiting that control to yourself through natural biofeedback are quite simple, including the positive body language messages you send to yourself while doing the exercises in this book. Other useful techniques are:

- *Learn pacing.* Don't take on too many obligations for the amount of time and energy you have available to devote to them.
- *Learn to say no.*
- *Learn to assert yourself* when it comes to getting what you need to take care of yourself.
- *Get enough sleep.*
- *Allow enough time for relaxation techniques.*
- *Allow sufficient exercise time for gentle muscle stretching.*
- Make sure you are getting *proper nourishment.* (See Resources.)
- *Decrease or eliminate your intake of stress-inducing substances,* including cocaine, marijuana, caffeine, tobacco, alcohol, and prescription drugs, especially analgesics, tranquilizers, antidepressants, sleeping pills, diet pills, and muscle relaxants. (Be sure to consult your physician before reducing or discontinuing any prescription medications. Ask your doctor to help you develop a schedule for decreasing your drug intake safely.)

In making all of these changes, you are exercising control over important aspects of your life, which will contribute to your health and well-being as well as to the proper functioning of your back.

Yoga Techniques for Coping With Stress
The Relaxation Response

Although most people feel that their leisure activities are relaxing, therapeutic relaxation means practicing a set of skills that create a specific physiological response. This response is not difficult to learn, but most Westerners have to be taught it, because it is not part of our cultural heritage.

The common denominator of all inducers of the relaxation response is an internal focus. Every time the mind wanders (and it will), bring your attention gently back to the focus point. Directing attention internally is the physiological opposite of directing attention to the outside world looking for danger. When attention is directed inward, your body receives messages that you are safe and secure and that it is appropriate to relax. So muscles relax, blood pressure drops, nerves are calmed, anxiety is decreased, immunity is heightened, and healing is enhanced.

The Relaxation Breath

A number of techniques can be used to create the relaxation response. My favorite is the Relaxation Breath taught by my yoga teacher, B.K.S. Iyengar. (Others include mechanical biofeedback, progressive muscular relaxation, guided imagery, Transcendental Meditation, and other types of meditation.)

The following Relaxation Breath is elegantly simple, yet quickly and effectively produces deep relaxation. It can be practiced either sitting or lying down.

Step 1. Inhale naturally through your nose.

Step 2. Exhale naturally through your nose.

Step 3. Pause while counting to yourself, one thousand one, one thousand two.

Step 4. Repeat steps 1, 2, and 3. Continue breathing in this manner for several minutes.

At the end of each exhalation, pause for a second or two before inhaling again. You may notice a spontaneous, unforced continuation of the exhalation during this pause. This additional release of breath completes a true normal exhalation.

If possible, breathe through your nose, but, of course, if your nose is congested, you must breathe through your mouth.

Do not try to inhale deeply, exhale deeply, or breathe slowly. If you feel the urge to inhale more deeply, follow this urge and then return to normal breathing.

Whenever possible, keep your eyes closed and looking down, as if they were looking at your lower eyelids. Notice how the eyes tend to look up with each inhalation. Resist this tendency. Notice the effect of your eye position on your awareness, calmness, and ability to relax. (If contact lenses make it uncomfortable to look down, look straight ahead; just don't allow your eyes to look up.)

Most people habitually exhale incompletely, starting each inhalation without allowing the previous exhalation to come to its natural conclusion. During one of my visits to his yoga institute in Pune, India, B.K.S. Iyengar explained to me that this incomplete exhalation provides "the soil, or base, for thought to arise." The mind jumps from one thought to another, the second thought arising before the first thought is ended, just as the inhalation begins before the exhalation is completed. If exhalation is allowed to conclude spontaneously and naturally, the mind does not have a chance to become agitated. When your awareness is repeatedly returned to the breathing process, the physiology of stress gives way to the relaxation response.

To facilitate learning, record the instructions for the Relaxation Breath on a cassette tape. Speak slowly, soothingly, and calmly to yourself. Remind yourself to relax your jaw muscles and keep your closed eyes looking down as you inhale and as you exhale. Play the tape when you practice the relaxation response, until you no longer need it.

If you already know another relaxation technique that works for you, fine! Keep on using it whenever you can and whenever it is called for in the exercise program. In addition to the Relaxation Breath, I use guided relaxations, focusing on watching the breath. I have recorded several of these guided relaxations on audiocassette for home use (see Resources).

Informal Practice of Relaxation Skills

Any number of daily activities can serve as your signal to practice the Relaxation Breath. You can practice it:

- At a stoplight
- Standing in an elevator
- Standing in line
- Waiting for an appointment
- Whenever you look at your watch
- Whenever you go to the bathroom
- Just before you pick up the telephone

There are a hundred times during the day in which a short relaxation break can bring you back to peace and equanimity. Each of these breaks allows you to release accumulated tensions so they don't build up into a full-blown stress response or, worse, a back attack. The following are a couple of ideas for relaxation breaks. Be creative! Invent your own relaxation breaks to fit your life.

- Massage your scalp, temples, and jaw. Focus on feeling the skin, muscles, and bones. Use your fingers to inform yourself about the tension in the muscles.

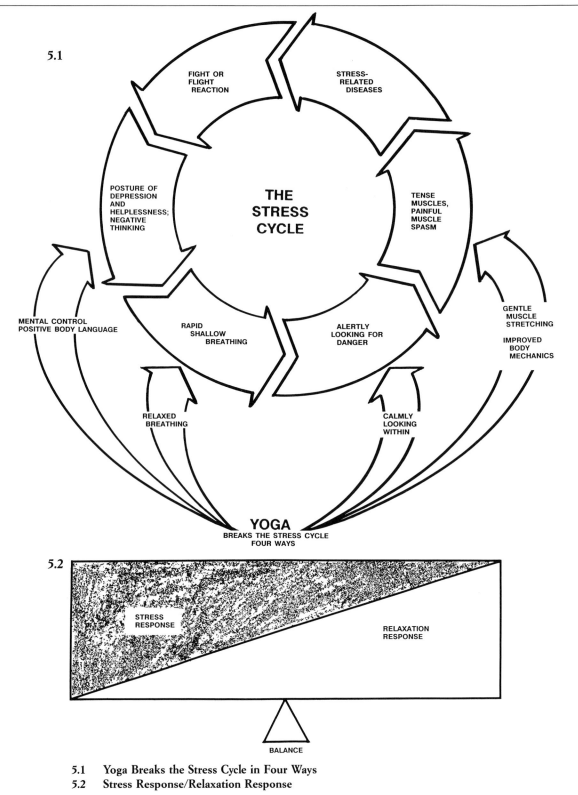

5.1 Yoga Breaks the Stress Cycle in Four Ways
5.2 Stress Response/Relaxation Response

First release the jaw muscles. Then let all these muscles go and feel the effects on your mental state.

• While brushing your teeth, slow down. Allow yourself to feel each brushstroke on your gums. Bring your attention to the here and now, away from thoughts about what is to come.

Formal Practice of the Relaxation Response

The relaxation response should be practiced daily as an unfailing component of your exercise routine. Practicing it at the end of your yoga sequence allows you to consciously release any muscle tension that may have built up. It also allows the new lessons of body carriage, strength, and flexibility to be absorbed by your nervous system and musculoskeletal system. Visualizing your posture improving and your back healing during formal relaxation is beneficial to the healing process.

During relaxation the spinal muscles lengthen, allowing greater separation of the vertebrae. This releases compression of the discs, allowing them to take in nourishment more efficiently.

The physiological state produced by the relaxation response enhances healing. It is the physiological opposite of the stress response, in which body tissues are broken down to provide energy for fight or flight (Figure 5.2).

Resting and Relaxing Your Back

Therapeutic, constructive rest is important in back rehabilitation. You may usually think of a resting position as being reclining or semireclining, but these positions can be harmful to a recovering back. Lounge chairs and soft sofas are frequent culprits. An example of destructive rest is the couch potato syndrome: lying with the spine rounded for hours, munching on snacks. Back pain can result in such situations from prolonged inactivity, poor posture, and weight gain.

In contrast, resting in restorative yoga poses allows the following:

• Support of the body in a position of good alignment, in which tired, overworked muscles can completely relax.
• Gentle, passive stretch for tight or overworked muscles.
• Correction of some asymmetries in muscle length and tension.
• Elimination of accumulated mental or emotional stresses and tensions.
• A repertoire of "positions of comfort" that you can use whenever you need them.

The Relaxation poses described in this chapter are a good way to start doing yoga. Practice one or more of them every day, following the routines suggested at the end of this chapter. After you have begun to practice the Home Base poses in Chapter 6, you can decrease the number of resting poses to one or two at the end of your sessions. It is also a good idea to do one or two resting poses before bedtime.

Practice Relaxation poses when you feel tired or when you become aware that your posture has slipped into old habits during any activity. These poses can also help you get the kinks out after a long trip or after mild trauma.

It is especially useful to practice Relaxation poses before commencing an activity that is likely to challenge your back. The postures can help you begin the potentially dangerous activity with a better alignment, so injury is less likely to occur. They can remind your muscles and bones of alignment principles, so you are more likely to use proper body mechanics as you pass through the danger zone. Afterward they can help you return to correct alignment. They may be used as a prelude and postlude to any vigorous activity, including sexual intercourse.

Try each resting pose and discover which ones are the most relaxing for you. If time is limited, use the two or three that work best, rather than going through a full routine.

To practice Relaxation poses, choose a place where you will be neither too warm nor too cold. Lying on a folded quilt or blanket on the floor (rather than on a bed) is best. Be sure to use good body mechanics while getting down onto the floor and coming back up (Figure 12.7). From a standing position, firmly place one foot slightly behind the other. Using a cane or a sturdy piece of furniture as needed for support, go down on one knee, keeping your ears over your center of gravity. Then kneel on both knees. Take your buttocks back toward your heels and sit to the side of your feet. To lie down, use your arms to ease one side of your torso down to the floor; then roll onto your back. To stand, reverse this process. If the pressure of the floor on your spine, sacrum, or tailbone is uncomfortable, put an extra folded towel or blanket under the tender spot.

Make sure that you will not be disturbed. You will not be able to relax fully if you know that you may have to pop up to answer the phone at any moment. If you do not have an answering machine, take the phone off the hook. Let the world wait.

If the room is cool or you have a tendency to become chilled, dress warmly and have a blanket nearby. Part of the physiological response to relaxation is the opening of the blood capillaries in the skin. This creates a transient warming feeling on the skin, which is followed by chilling, as the blood loses heat to the surrounding cool air through the dilated capillaries.

Supporting the Head and Neck

Remember that the natural curve of the neck is convex toward the front and concave toward the back. Deep relaxation and release of muscle tension in the neck and shoulders is greatly facilitated by proper support of the cervical curve and the back of the head with carefully selected padding.

The support for the back of the neck must be firm, not soft and compressible. Rolled or folded towels and bath mats work quite well.

Before proceeding further, take the time to work out your neck and head padding. Do not shortchange yourself by rushing through this section. The benefits of proper neck and head padding will be worth more than you can imagine. Your time will be well rewarded with relaxation, comfort, and pain relief. Conscientious attention to neck and head padding is especially important for those who have upper back or neck discomfort.

Preparing the Neck Support Rolls

Assemble four hand towels. You will make several different-sized rolls to try. Carefully fold one towel in half and smoothly roll it (no wrinkles allowed) into a roll four inches in diameter. Secure it with rubber bands. Fold another towel in thirds and roll it to a diameter of approximately six inches. Fold the last two towels in half, place one on top of the other, and roll them together to form a thicker roll, about eight inches in diameter. Secure each roll with one or two rubber bands.

Preparing the Head Pads

Assemble four bath towels. To prepare the pads to put behind your head, carefully fold each towel to a thickness of two, four, six, or eight inches, and secure each pad with a couple of pieces of tape. Be sure that the pad has no lumps in it.

Trying Out the Rolls and Pads

If your alignment evaluation from the side (Figure 4.12) showed that you had good alignment of the head over the shoulders, with the centers of the ears over the centers of the shoulder joints, begin with the thinnest head pad and the smallest roll. If your evaluation showed that your head is significantly forward, start with the middle thicknesses.

Place a roll under your neck and a pad under your head. The roll should be low on the neck, perpendicular to the spine, with one long edge touching the tops of the shoulders. Lie on your back with your knees bent, and experience the feeling of this combination (Figure 5.3).

Then try out the next larger roll and pad. See how that feels and compare it with the first one. Experiment with the thicknesses of the rolls and pads until you find the combination that feels the best.

You should feel support and comfort behind the neck, but your throat should not feel compressed (padding too thick, Figure 5.4). Nor should the throat feel overstretched (padding too thin, Figure 5.5). If the thickest diameter roll and the thickest pad feel best for you, try a slightly larger roll and a slightly thicker pad to see if you need even more support.

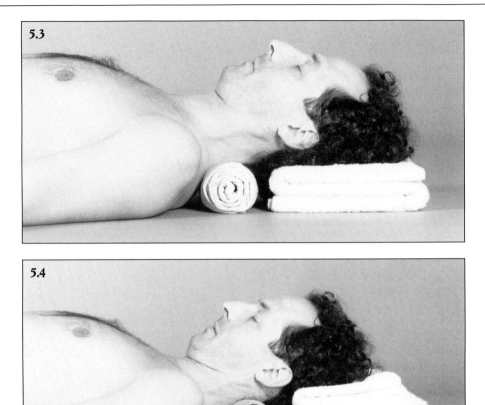

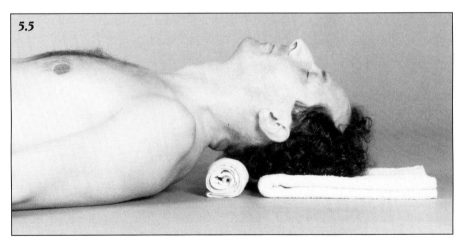

5.3   Head Pad and Neck Support Roll, Correct Position
5.4   Head Pad and Neck Support Roll, Too Thick
5.5   Head Pad and Neck Support Roll, Too Thin

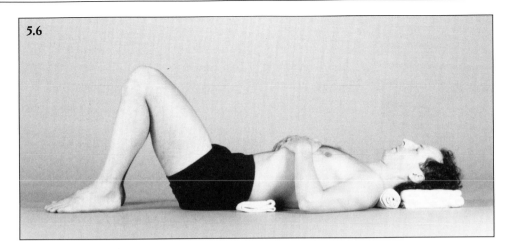

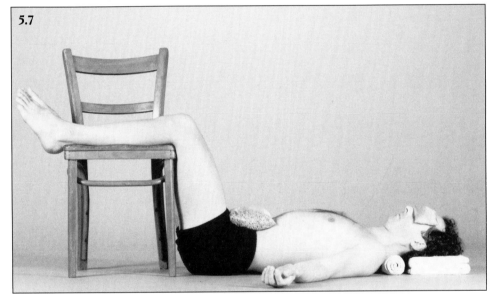

5.6   **Lumbar Pad Placement**
5.7   **Lying Down with Calves on Chair**

Once you have chosen the perfect set of roll and pad, secure them with tape and slip them in a pillow case. Always have them handy when you are doing yoga. You may also enjoy using them while sleeping.

Lumbar Pad

If you have a flat lumbar curve, make a lumbar pad by folding a bath towel like a closed fan so that it is between a half an inch and an inch thick and the folds are three to four inches wide. Use this every time a lumbar pad is called for. Place it where it feels best—start with it just behind the waist, and then move it down toward the pelvis until it feels right (Figure 5.6). You may need to experiment with different thicknesses to find the perfect one for your lumbar support. If the lumbar pad doesn't seem to work for you, leave it out for now and try it again in a few months.

About the Yoga Poses

The yoga poses in this book are presented in a format that ensures you will understand exactly how to proceed. The section labeled "Props needed" will let you know which props to have close at hand. The props listed in parentheses may not be needed by everyone. "Position and Adjustment" tells you how to get into the pose and how to modify it for your personal needs. This section will also tell you how long to stay in the pose and how many times to repeat it.

"Breathing and Imagery" instructions will remind you how to breathe in the pose. Using the suggested imagery will help you automatically assume the proper alignment without consciously placing every bone and muscle.

The "Rationale" section explains the specific purpose of each pose and the benefits that you will receive from it. "Notes" at the end of each exercise provide tips for those with special conditions such as pregnancy or spondylolisthesis.

✣

Lying Down with Calves on a Chair

Props needed: chair, neck support roll, head pad,
two- to four-pound weight (such as a bag of rice or
dried beans). (As needed: lumbar pad, cloth or
eyebag.)

Position and Adjustment. Lie on your back, with your calves resting on a chair seat, sofa, or other prop of an appropriate height so that your knees and your hips are bent at about ninety degrees. Place the weight on your abdomen between your waist and your pubic bone (Figure 5.7).

Make sure that your neck support roll and head pad are appropriately placed and of the proper thickness to comfortably support your spine. (Use your lumbar pad if you have a flat lumbar curve.) You may wish to place a cloth or an eyebag (see Resources) over your eyes.

Slide your hands behind your waist and then down under your buttocks toward your legs. This will release any tension in the lumbar area by readjusting the buttock skin and flesh. Then roll your shoulders back and under, so that your arms rest comfortably with the palms facing up.

Rest here for one to five minutes. Then roll onto your side and rest there for thirty to sixty seconds before using your arms to push yourself to a seated position. Move quietly to the next pose.

Breathing and Imagery. Use the Relaxation Breath, pausing at the end of each exhalation. Keep your eyes closed and looking down, as if they were looking at your lower eyelids. Visualize your spine's normal curves being supported by the props and the floor.

Rationale. This supported Relaxation pose is especially effective for resting the lower back and shoulders. The weight on the abdomen creates a pleasant feeling of release and relaxation in the muscles and nerves of the spine.

Notes

- *This is a good pose for those with spondylolysis or spondylolisthesis.*
- *Do not use the weight on your abdomen if you are pregnant.*
- *Do not practice this pose during the second half of pregnancy.*

❧

Elbows on the Table

Props needed: chair, table.

Position and Adjustment. Sit in a straight chair on a nonslip surface in front of a table, so that you can comfortably lean forward onto the table. Rest your head and folded arms on the table (Figure 5.8). Avoid letting your lower back overarch. Soften your front lower ribs back into your body to slightly flatten the lumbar curve and stretch the paraspinal muscles (the muscles on either side of the spine). Hold this position for twenty to thirty seconds, breathing normally. Release and repeat several times, alternating the crossed position of the arms. (If you begin with the left forearm on top, place the right forearm on top the next time, and so on.) Always return to the erect sitting position slowly, breathing deeply, to avoid dizziness.

Breathing and Imagery. With each breath, allow your lower back to lengthen and release. Use the Relaxation Breath, breathing normally and pausing at the end of each exhalation for several seconds.

Rationale. This supported position allows the spinal muscles to release and lengthen so that the vertebrae can separate and allow the discs to expand. Resting the forehead in this way encourages the relaxation response by relieving the neck and shoulder muscles of their burden.

Notes

- *If you have a flat lumbar curve, allow your lower back to arch slightly toward a more normal curve.*
- *This pose is not suitable for those with spondylolysis, spondylolisthesis, or posterior or lateral bulging discs.*
- *This is a great back rester for those in late pregnancy.*

❊

Chair-Seated Forward Bend
with Torso Support

Props needed: two chairs, four to six blankets.
(As needed: thick towel.)

Position and Adjustment. Fold each blanket in half lengthwise, then fanfold it to create a rectangular support twelve inches wide. Stack the blankets neatly and place them across the seat of one of the chairs, so that the long side of the stack is parallel with the back of the chair. (If you have yoga bolsters, they can be used instead. See Resources.)

Sit in the other chair facing the side of the first chair. Separate your knees and pull the blanketed chair between your legs so that you are looking out over the long axis of the folded pile of blankets. Stretch your torso up as tall as is comfortably possible. Using your arms for support, lower your torso onto the pile of blankets (Figure 5.9). If possible, allow your forehead to rest on the blankets or turn your head to one side and rest there for several minutes. If your head does not reach the blankets, fold the towel and place it under your head. Increase or decrease the thickness of the chest support by adding or taking away blankets until you are comfortable. Allow your abdominal muscles to become soft and passive. Release your back with each exhalation.

To come up, use the support of your arms to push your torso back up to a seated position, keeping your abdominal and paraspinal muscles relaxed. (It is very important to use your arms, not your paraspinal muscles, to lift out of the pose: Otherwise your paraspinal muscles might go into spasm.) Move quietly to the next pose.

Breathing and Imagery. Inhale and exhale normally. Pause briefly at the end of each exhalation to allow further spontaneous release of the breath. Allow your abdomen to gently expand with each inhalation. See the muscles of your back relaxing and releasing tightness and spasm. See your spine elongating. See pain and fatigue escaping the body with every exhalation.

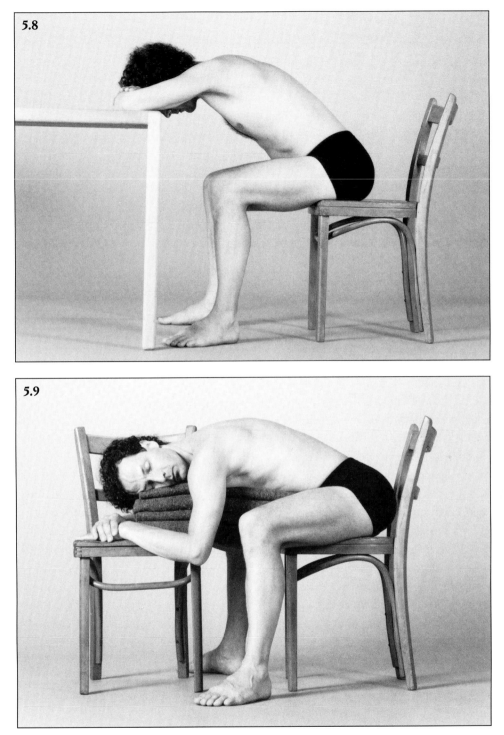

5.8   Elbows on the Table
5.9   Chair-Seated Forward Bend with Torso Support

Rationale. With the abdomen relaxed and the torso supported, the back muscles can relax and lengthen, allowing more space between the vertebrae for better disc nourishment and healing.

Notes

- *This pose is not suitable for those with spondylolysis or spondylolisthesis.*
- *Do not practice this pose during the second half of pregnancy.*

Supine Child's Pose

Props needed: neck support roll, head pad.
(As needed: lumbar pad.)

Position and Adjustment. Lie on your back with your knees bent, and the neck support roll and head pad in the proper positions. Use your lumbar pad, if needed, for flat back.

Draw your knees toward your chest and hold them in a comfortable position. To avoid compression of the knees, hold the backs of the thighs, not the shins (Figure 5.10).

Inhale, and on the next exhalation, slowly draw your thighs toward your chest until your buttocks are lifted slightly from the floor.

Inhale and gently let your buttocks back down to the floor, slightly further away from your head than when you started.

Stay in this position, watching your breathing, for one to three minutes. Then rest on one side for thirty to sixty seconds before sitting. Move quietly to the next pose.

Breathing and Imagery. As you breathe, using the Relaxation Breath, imagine that your back is getting longer and that the muscles along the sides of the spine are becoming relaxed. See a new, more natural lumbar curve being created as the result of relaxing and breathing in this position.

Rationale. This pose stretches and relaxes the paraspinal muscles while the floor supports the weight of the body.

Notes

- *This is an excellent Relaxation pose for spondylolysis and spondylolisthesis, as it uses position and gravity to reduce the tendency for the vertebrae to slip forward.*
- *Do not practice this pose during the second half of pregnancy.*

Child's Pose

Props needed: pad. (As needed: two twisted socks, rolled towel, folded blanket.)

Position and Adjustment. Kneel and rest your chest on your thighs. Place your forehead on the floor or turn your head to one side. For comfort you can place a pad under your knees or your head, or both (Figure 5.11). If you can't get your head on the floor, use a folded blanket of the proper height for head support. If your knees hurt, you can place a twisted sock in the bend of each knee to create more space. A rolled towel under your ankles can relieve excessive stretch there. If your buttocks don't rest on your heels, place a folded blanket on your lower legs and sit on that (Figure 5.12).

Breathing and Imagery. Inhale into your abdomen and back. On each exhalation, release your spine and visualize it getting longer. As you go through several breath cycles, your trunk will actually passively elongate. To accommodate this elongation, lift your chest and abdomen off your thighs slightly, accept the new length, and rest again on your thighs. Stay here as long as you can, up to several minutes. Keep relaxing and lengthening into the pose. Sit up slowly, using the arms to support the trunk. Move quietly to the next pose.

Rationale. This is a relaxing passive stretch for the muscles on either side of the spine. It teaches conscious relaxation of these muscles, which can stay tense without your being aware of it, and helps reeducate them to have a longer resting length. This allows more space between the vertebrae for the discs and decreases disc degeneration caused by constant compression.

Notes

- *It is important to use the strength of your arms to push up to a sitting position. Otherwise, your newly relaxed paraspinal muscles might go into painful spasm.*
- *If this posture bothers your knees, do Chair-Seated Forward Bend with Torso Support (Figure 5.9) instead.*
- *This is not a recommended position for those with spondylolysis, spondylolisthesis, or posterior or lateral bulging discs. If you have spondylolysis or spondylolisthesis, this and other forward bends can actually aggravate the tendency for forward slippage of the damaged vertebra. Therefore, substitute Supine Child's Pose (Figure 5.10).*
- *This pose can be practiced in the first half of pregnancy if the knees are separated widely to accommodate the growing baby and the belly is not compressed against the floor. During the second half of pregnancy, practice this pose only as long as you can do so without compressing the abdomen.*

✿
Chair-Seated Twist with Torso Support

Props needed: two chairs, three to six blankets, towel.

Position and Adjustment. Place the chairs side by side on a nonskid surface. Sit on one chair and place a neatly folded pile of blankets lengthwise on the chair next to you, just as you did for Chair-Seated Forward Bend with Torso Support. (If you have yoga bolsters, they can be used instead. See Resources.) Make sure that your feet are either on the floor or supported by several books so that they do not dangle. Inhale. On the next exhalation, stretch your arms above your head and lengthen your torso upward. Turn your torso to face the blankets. Place your hands on the blankets and use the strength of your arms to lower your torso onto them (Figure 5.13).

If this action causes uncomfortable stretch on the side of the body that started out farthest from the pile of blankets, then you may need a higher support for your trunk. Try adding another neatly folded blanket. If there is discomfort in the hip or back on the side next to the chair, come out of the pose and start over. This time, take care not to collapse that side, but keep it lengthening, as you lower your torso.

Rest there for several breaths. Allow the outer hip (the hip that started out farther from the blankets) to feel heavy and to move down passively toward the chair seat as you release your muscles to the stretch. Before coming up from the pose, visualize yourself getting up. Then slowly place your hands beneath your shoulders and use the strength of your arms to push yourself back up into a sitting position, to avoid asking the softened, stretched, and relaxed back muscles to contract and pull you upright.

To stretch the other side, switch places with the blankets. Maintain quietness and relaxation. Don't allow your consciousness to become agitated as you change position. Keep your eyes looking down, as if you are looking at your lower eyelids. Stay deeply relaxed during this transition, so that as you go down onto the blankets again, you begin with the same depth of relaxation that you had previously achieved.

Do this stretch for several breaths on each side. One side will usually be easier to do. If your paraspinal muscles are in spasm, repeat this pose six times on each side, alternating from one side to the other. Notice how your back responds to the gentle persistence of the repetitions by letting go of tightness and discomfort.

Breathing and Imagery. Continue using the Relaxation Breath. Imagine that you are breathing into the area where you feel the most stretch. Imagine that each breath is elongating the area along the side of the spine toward the hip. Visualize this area as a long balloon that is becoming gradually inflated with each breath.

Rationale. This pose helps relieve spasm and correct asymmetry in lengths of the muscles on either side of the back. It is wonderful for times when the paraspinal muscles are in spasm, because each repetition allows them to release and relax.

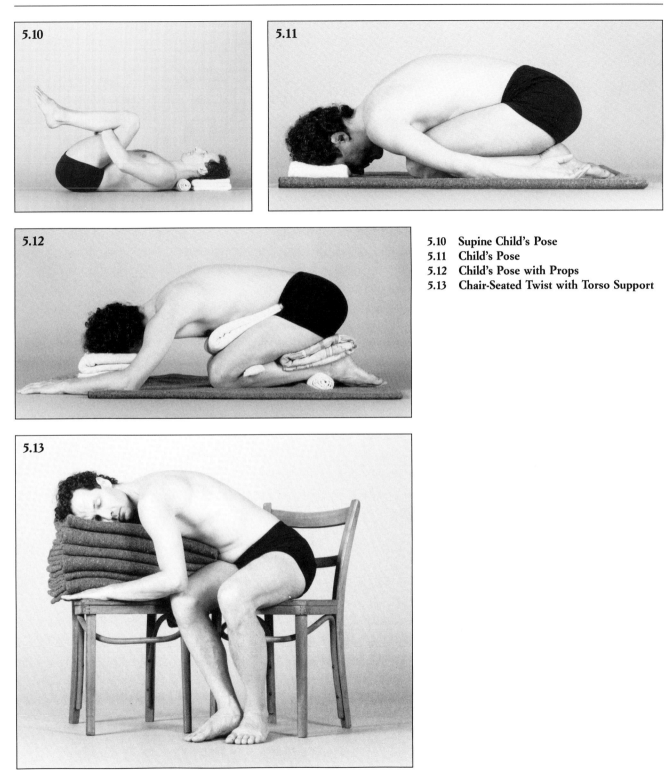

5.10   **Supine Child's Pose**
5.11   **Child's Pose**
5.12   **Child's Pose with Props**
5.13   **Chair-Seated Twist with Torso Support**

Note

• *Do not practice this pose during the second half of pregnancy.*

❧

Supine Resting with Knee Support

Props needed: neck support roll, head pad, rolled
blanket, two- to four-pound weight (such as a bag of
rice or dried beans). (As needed: lumbar pad,
folded towel.)

Position and Adjustment. Lie on your back on the floor, legs extended. Position the neck support roll and head pad. Place the rolled blanket behind your knees. Slide your hands beneath your buttocks toward your knees to release your lumbar spine (Figure 5.14). If you have a flat lumbar curve, use your lumbar pad.

If your tailbone or sacrum is uncomfortable, put an additional folded towel under the tender spot. Place the weight on your abdomen between your waist and your pubic bone. Roll your shoulders back and under so that your palms face the ceiling and your arms are slightly away from your sides. Close your eyes.

Breathing and Imagery. Use the Relaxation Breath. Release your body into the floor and be aware of its heaviness. Allow your neck, upper back, lumbar spine, sacrum, and head to be fully supported by the floor and the props. With each exhalation, continue to surrender your weight more completely to the floor. In your mind's eye, see the muscles along either side of your spine releasing and letting go. Mentally connect this releasing of your muscles to your breathing and imagery. As you inhale, imagine that your spine is elongating, just as an accordion does when the two ends are pulled apart. As you exhale, maintain this increased length. On the next inhalation, breathe your spine even longer. Remember to keep your eyes closed and looking down toward your lower eyelids. (If this seems to strain your eyes, your head pad may not be thick enough.) Keep a blanket nearby in case you get chilled.

Stay in this position for two to ten minutes. When you are ready to come out of the pose, roll onto one side, and pause there before using the strength of your arms to push yourself up into a seated position.

Rationale. The floor and the props support your weight, allowing your muscles to relax. The blanket behind your knees releases the pull of the hip flexors on the pelvis and lumbar vertebrae and prevents the knees from hyperextending. The weight on the abdomen encourages rapid relaxation of the abdominal muscles and hip flexors and facilitates release of the paraspinal muscles.

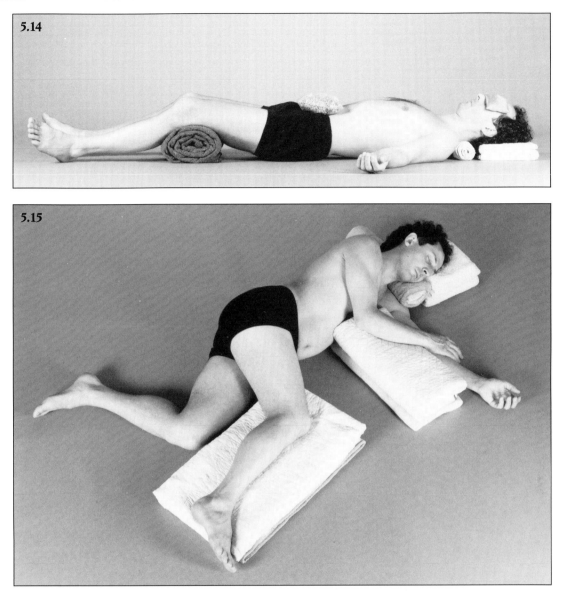

5.14   **Supine Resting with Knee Support**
5.15   **Side-Lying Relaxation**

Notes

- *Do not use the weight if you are pregnant.*
- *Do not practice this pose during the second half of pregnancy.*

❧

Side-Lying Relaxation

Props needed: head pad, neck support roll,
two blankets.

Position and Adjustment. Lie on your side, with the lower leg straight and the upper leg bent. Arrange the head pad and neck support roll. The head pad should be thick enough to fill the space between the floor, the side of your head and neck, and the top of your shoulder. (Note: This will be thicker than the support needed for the head and neck when lying on your back.) Place your upper knee and upper arm on the folded blankets (Figure 5.15). Elongate the sides of your body by stretching each hip in turn away from your lower ribs.

Breathing and Imagery. Use the Relaxation Breath. Continue to breathe your spine long with each inhalation and exhalation. Keep your eyes closed, looking down at your lower eyelids.

Stay here for two to ten minutes or as long as you are comfortable. Keep a blanket handy in case you get chilled. Return to sitting slowly, to avoid dizziness.

Rationale. This is a resting pose for those who are uncomfortable lying on their backs. It is also a great sleeping position.

Note

- *This is the best resting pose for the latter half of pregnancy (see Figure 11.13). A pillow can be placed under the belly for additional support and comfort.*

Suggested Routines

Five Minutes

Flat Back or Normal Back
1. Supine Child's Pose (Figure 5.10)
2. Lying Down with Calves on a Chair (Figure 5.7)

Swayback or Normal Back
1. Child's Pose (Figure 5.11)
2. Lying Down with Calves on a Chair (Figure 5.7)

Pregnancy
1. Elbows on the Table (Figure 5.8)
2. Child's Pose, knees separated (Figure 5.11)
3. Side-Lying Relaxation (Figure 11.13)

Fifteen Minutes

Routine A
1. Chair-Seated Forward Bend with Torso Support, two minutes (Figure 5.9)
2. Chair-Seated Twist with Torso Support, four minutes (Figure 5.13)
3. Child's Pose, four minutes (Figure 5.11)
4. Lying Down with Calves on a Chair, five minutes (Figure 5.7)

Routine B
1. Lying Down with Calves on a Chair, four minutes (Figure 5.7)
2. Supine Child's Pose, three minutes (Figure 5.10)
3. Child's Pose, three minutes (Figure 5.11)
4. Supine Resting with Knee Support, five minutes (Figure 5.14)

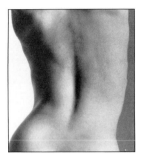

Six

Home Base Poses

*B*ack rehabilitation must be approached with love and respect for your body and a growing faith in its ability to improve. The following chapters present yoga exercises that can dramatically transform your back. This program should be practiced with a nonaggressive state of mind. You must acknowledge the necessity for slow, steady change in order to reform your alignment, body tissues, and self-image. Remember that back injuries are usually cumulative, resulting from years, or even decades, of injurious posture and movements. Patience and diligence will be rewarded with slow, steady improvement.

For your exercise sessions, wear clothes that allow you to see your alignment. Remember Thoreau's advice: "Beware of all enterprises that require new clothes." There is no need to acquire a wardrobe of high fashion leotards and tights—a pair of loose shorts and a T-shirt will work just fine. The feet *must* be bare to allow observation of alignment and to keep you from slipping. Avoid long pants with baggy legs, which prevent you from observing ankle and knee alignment and leg muscle function.

Besides your head and neck support rolls and lumbar pad, useful props to have on hand are blankets and a nonskid yoga mat (if you don't have a nonskid floor surface) to keep your feet from slipping (see Resources). You will feel more comfortable doing the exercises if you have not eaten for two to four hours before you practice (two hours after a light meal, four hours after a heavy meal). But do not let this guideline become an excuse for not practicing. It is better to practice with a slightly uncomfortable feeling in your abdomen than to skip your exercises and allow your back to deteriorate. Once your body learns how much better it feels when you wait the proper amount of time after eating, it will be easier for you to arrange your schedule.

I am frequently asked when the best time is to practice yoga. Only you can answer this question. When does it best fit into your day? Are you an early bird or a night owl? As you experiment with practicing at different times, you might find that you prefer to do more active poses in the morning and more relaxing poses in the evening—or vice versa. Decide for yourself. Don't let your preconceptions about when you should practice become a barrier to practicing at all.

Be Your Own Yoga Teacher

Using a tape recorder can free you from having to read and do yoga poses at the same time. I remember how clumsy and inept I felt trying to do poses while holding my first yoga book open with my foot so I could read the instructions. If you use a tape recorder, you won't find yourself wishing that you had a third arm or leg. (See Resources for information on audiocassettes I have recorded for home use.)

To use the tape recorder to become your own yoga teacher, begin by reading completely through the instructions for an exercise and then practicing it. Read through once again and practice again. In this way you will discover which of the instructions pertain to you, and you can record only the ones you need. Speak slowly to give yourself time to perform the movements and adjustments that are called for. Keep your voice calm and relaxed, so that those feelings will influence your performance of the pose.

Don't worry if the tape isn't perfect. The erase button is always there! In fact, it would be unusual for your first recordings to remain what you need later on in your practice.

Add new poses, one at a time, to create your own personal yoga routine.

How To Practice

Give yourself *several months* practicing just the Home Base poses in this chapter. Then, every two weeks or so, add one Moving On pose from Chapter 7 and practice it along with your Home Base exercises. It is important to end each practice session with one or two poses from Chapter 5, "Relaxation Techniques." If you have a special condition (such as scoliosis or sciatica) that is given a separate chapter in this book, alternate your Home Base routines and your "special condition" routines for several months. Then gradually begin adding Moving On poses.

Proceeding gradually can help prevent discouragement and setbacks due to overexertion or incorrect practice. (If a setback occurs or you lapse in your practice, see "Setbacks" and "Backsliding" in Chapter 3.) Plan to spend fifteen to thirty minutes, five or six days a week, on these poses. Give yourself one day a week off in which you practice only poses from Chapter 5, "Relaxation Techniques."

At the end of each practice chapter are several timed routines. Choose a routine based on how much time you have available—or invent your own, being sure to end with a Relaxation pose. Remember that the more you practice, the more your back will improve—still, it's better to do just a little bit than to skip your yoga entirely because you don't have enough time. When time is short, just do one pose well for a minute or two—and feel good about it.

How To Breathe in Yoga Poses

Proper breathing is essential to achieve maximum benefit from yoga poses. When you are in danger, your breathing becomes rapid and shallow, sending signals that you are in danger to the stress-monitoring parts of the brain. Muscles automatically tense up. On the other hand, when your breathing is relaxed and quiet, the brain receives messages of stability and well-being, and the physiology of the body shifts away from emergency reactions and toward the relaxation response.

Therefore it is important to breathe well in the yoga poses. Inhale and exhale through your nose. (Do not inhale through the nose and exhale through the mouth, as is taught in some relaxation courses.) If your nose is congested, then, of course, you must breathe through your mouth.

The sounds of the breath should not be audible to someone standing near you. Noisy breathing is interpreted by the brain as a sign of stress. Also, breathing during yoga exercises should not be restricted in any way. (In some of the more sophisticated yogic breathing techniques, part of the throat is closed off while breathing. However, these techniques should be practiced only after studying with an experienced teacher.)

For breathing during yoga exercises, the basic rule is that as you inhale, you do nothing except focus on your posture while relaxing the muscles of the face, jaw, and shoulders. With the exhalation, perform the action of the pose. (Any exceptions to this basic rule will be noted in the instructions for the poses.)

Trying to attend to specific patterns of breathing can be unnecessarily confusing for beginners. The most important thing is to keep breathing quietly and naturally. Never hold your breath!

Focusing on your breathing while doing yoga adds a meditative aspect to your exercise. Meditation involves keeping your awareness on a single thought, sound, or body process, such as breathing. When you constantly return your wandering mind to the breath, the outside world recedes. Then the focus becomes internal, promoting relaxation and self-awareness, rather than external, promoting stress.

To stop them from keeping the abdomen rigid while breathing, yoga students are often instructed to "breathe into the belly." Unfortunately, some people have taken this to mean that you should breathe only with the belly and not with the chest. Not only is this almost impossible, but trying to breathe with the chest rigid is just as bad as trying to breathe with the abdomen rigid. It limits lung expansion and sends signals of stress to the brain.

Breathing well in the poses requires what I call "Total Torso Breathing." To experience this, try the following exercise. Kneel comfortably in Child's Pose (Figure 5.11) or bend forward and rest your torso on your thighs while sitting in a chair with a firm seat. Breathe normally and focus on the feelings of gentle expansion in the chest wall with each inhalation and exhalation. As you inhale, feel the front ribs press against the thighs. As you exhale, experience the change in the feelings of the skin of your chest.

On the next inhalation, imagine that you are inhaling into your belly. As you inhale, feel the ribs move as before, but also allow yourself to feel your belly expanding against your thighs. In order to do this, your abdominal wall muscles must be soft and relaxed. With each inhalation feel your chest expand, as well as your abdomen.

Now take your awareness to the pelvic diaphragm, the sheet of muscles that spans the space between the tailbone, the sitting bones, and the pubic bone. (These are the muscles that contract to control urination and bowel movements.) Inhale into your chest and abdomen, and in your mind's eye take your breath all the way to your pelvic diaphragm. Allow yourself to feel the pelvic diaphragm expanding outward on each inhalation, just as the chest and abdomen do. Continue breathing this way, focusing on breathing with your entire torso: the front chest, the back chest, the front and sides of the abdomen, and the pelvis. This is Total Torso Breathing.

Home Base Poses

The poses in this chapter provide both beginning and continuing yoga practitioners with the first steps in stretching tight muscles, strengthening weak muscles, and improving posture. Continuing students will find the Home Base poses useful for warming up before and cooling down after any type of vigorous exercise. They are also beneficial as a fall-back routine when your back feels tender or vulnerable.

When you begin to practice the Home Base poses, do so slowly, without forcing yourself or going faster than is absolutely comfortable. As you work with these postures, continue to use the relaxation techniques that you learned in Chapter 5.

Above all, approach the exercises with a positive, pleasant, explorative state of mind, expecting to enjoy doing something good for yourself.

❧

Supine Pelvic Tilt

Props needed: neck support roll, head pad.
(As needed: lumbar pad.)

Positions and Adjustment. Lie on your back with your knees bent and your feet parallel on the floor. Place your arms comfortably at your sides, palms up. Place your head pad under your head and your neck support roll under your neck.

Inhale into your chest and abdomen. Let your chest and belly expand. As you exhale, move your navel toward the floor. This action will take your lower back toward the floor as well (Figure 6.1). Inhale again into your abdomen; on an exhalation, again press your navel and lower back toward the floor. At the same time, press your shoulders, elbows, and the back of your head into the floor. Keep your legs entirely passive. Repeat slowly at least ten times. Work towards being able to hold the position for ten to twenty seconds. Roll to your side and then sit up.

Breathing and Imagery. See your spine assuming a more normal configuration. Explore the feelings in the muscles called on to produce this action. Realize that by pressing down with the shoulders and elbows you are keeping your shoulders from rounding and your chest from collapsing as you move your navel toward the floor.

Rationale. An important first step in reeducating your posture, this exercise teaches awareness of chest alignment and its relationship to the position of the pelvis and the lumbar spine. For those with a normal lumbar curve or with swayback, it teaches awareness of how your body responds to decreases of your lumbar curve. It also begins to strengthen the abdominal muscles, an important step in creating a healthy back no matter what type of spinal curve you have. For those with rounded shoulders or forward head posture, it provides gentle correction toward a healthier alignment.

Notes

- *If you have a flat back, do this pose with your lumbar pad in place.*
- *If you have spondylolysis or spondylolisthesis, this is an important pose for you.*
- *Do not practice this pose during the second half of pregnancy.*

❧

Yoga Sit-Ups

Props needed: chair. (As needed: lumbar pad.)

Position and Adjustment. Lie on your back with your calves resting on a chair seat. Your hips as well as your knees should be bent at about a ninety-degree angle. Cross your arms in front of your chest and place your hands on your shoulders (Figure 6.2). *To avoid neck strain, do not place your hands on your neck!* If you want more of a challenge, lightly hold each earlobe or cross your arms behind your head and touch each shoulder blade with the opposite hand (Figure 6.3). Again, do not place your hands on your neck.

Action, Breathing, and Imagery. Inhale. Begin a long, slow exhalation, during which you:

- Tilt the pelvis as described in the preceding pose, so your lower back moves to the floor as you flatten your abdomen
- Raise your shoulders six to ten inches off the floor, no higher
- Lower your right shoulder to touch the floor and raise it back up (Figure 6.4)
- Continue exhaling as you lower your trunk to the floor

Inhale; on a long, slow exhalation, repeat the preceding sequence, this time lowering and raising your left shoulder. Visualize your abdominal muscles getting stronger as you use them to lift your trunk. Repeat the sequence with proper breathing until your abdominal muscles feel warm. Then do one or two more and stop. Roll to the side and use the strength of your arms to push yourself into a seated position.

Caution. Do not hold your breath during any part of this exercise.

Rationale. Having the hips flexed at about ninety degrees prevents injury to the lumbar spine. Lifting the trunk while exhaling places the abdominals in a shortened position for strengthening, preventing you from ending up with strong but "puffed out" (protruding) abdominal muscles less capable of lumbar support. Lifting straight up strengthens the midline abdominal muscles. Lowering and lifting each shoulder strengthens the other abdominal muscles. The abdomen should not bulge out, but should feel flatter and wider during this exercise.

Safe strengthening of the abdominal muscles is crucial to proper positioning of the pelvis and maintenance of a healthy lumbar curve.

Notes

- *If you have a flat back, use your lumbar pad to create and support a more natural curve during this exercise.*
- *If you have spondylolysis or spondylolisthesis, this is another important pose for you.*
- *Do not practice this pose during the second half of pregnancy.*

❧

Supine Knee-Chest Twist

Props needed: neck support roll, head pad.

Position and Adjustment, Variation 1. Lie on your back with your neck support roll and head pad in place. Place your arms out to each side, palms up. Bend both knees and draw them toward your chest together. Inhale, and on the exhalation, let both

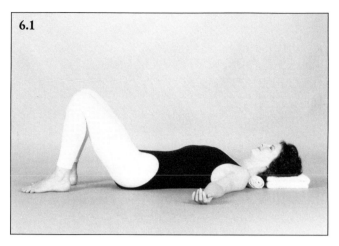

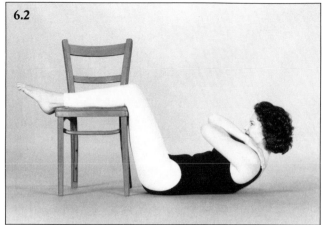

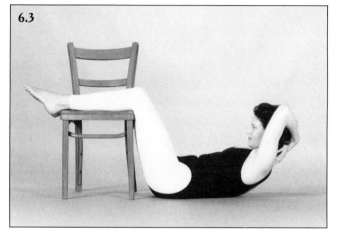

6.1   Supine Pelvic Tilt
6.2   Yoga Sit-Ups, Arms Crossed on Chest
6.3   Yoga Sit-Ups, Arms Crossed Behind Head
6.4   Yoga Sit-Ups, Lowering One Shoulder

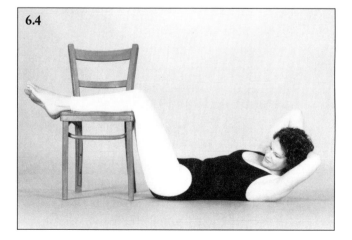

knees slowly and gently down to the floor on one side of your body (Figure 6.5). Rest them there for thirty to sixty seconds. Inhale, and on the exhalation, slowly lift your knees back to the starting position. Repeat on the other side. Do three to five sets.

Note

- *If you have spondylolysis or spondylolisthesis, do this first variation rather than the second.*

Variation 2. To intensify the strengthening aspects of this pose, slowly lower your knees to one side, stopping a few inches off the floor (or when the opposite shoulder begins to leave the floor). Press your elbows and shoulders into the floor to gain more control of your legs. Hold your legs there for three to ten seconds, breathing quietly (Figure 6.6). Don't hold your breath! On an exhalation, lift your knees, continuing to press your elbows and shoulders to the floor. Repeat on the other side. Do three to five sets.

Breathing and Imagery. Use the Relaxation Breath and Total Torso Breathing. Imagine your spine lengthening.

Rationale. These poses can be used to stretch the paraspinal muscles, as well as to strengthen the abdominal muscles. The abdominal muscles are called upon to stabilize the trunk as the legs are let down toward the floor, and to help lift the legs and turn the pelvis when returning to the starting position. The paraspinal muscles receive a gentle stretch while the legs are resting on the floor. Lengthening these muscles provides more space for disc nourishment and healing.

Notes

- *Do not practice these poses during the second half of pregnancy.*
- *If you experience pain or numbness in Variation 1 or 2, discontinue practicing this pose and refer to the "Begin with Caution" page at the front of the book.*

❧

Crocodile Twist

Props needed: head pad, neck support roll.

Position and Adjustment. Lie on your back with your head pad and neck support roll in place. Bend your right knee and place your right foot on top of your left knee. Roll over onto your left side, so that your right knee touches the floor. Use your left hand to stabilize your right knee on the floor (Figure 6.7). Lower your right shoulder away from your right ear. Then stretch your right arm toward the ceiling and back in an arc behind the body. Keep your left leg active by stretching out through the heel and pulling the toes back toward you. It is not important for your right hand to touch the floor. Stay here for several breaths (thirty to sixty seconds).

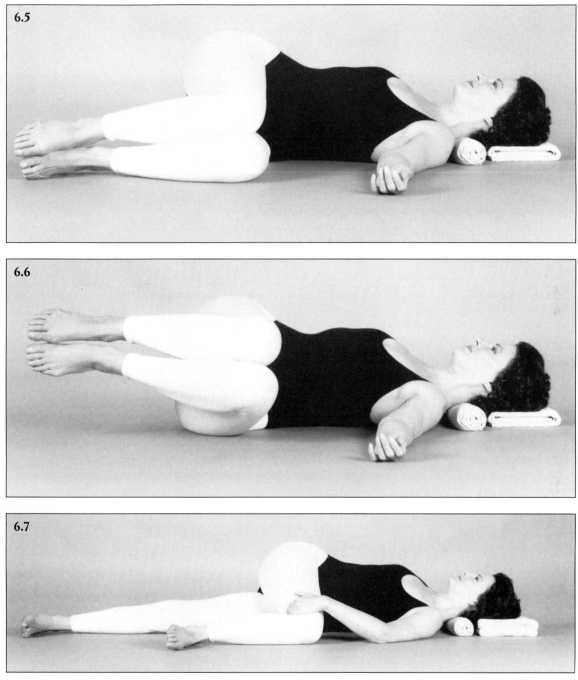

6.5   Supine Knee to Chest, Variation 1
6.6   Supine Knee to Chest, Variation 2
6.7   Crocodile Twist

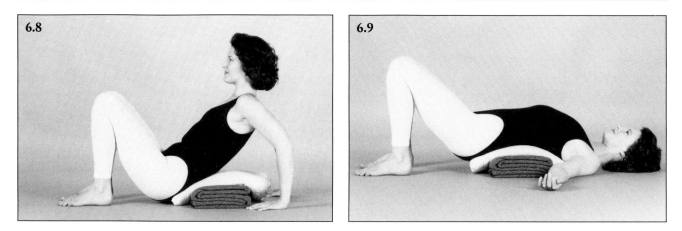

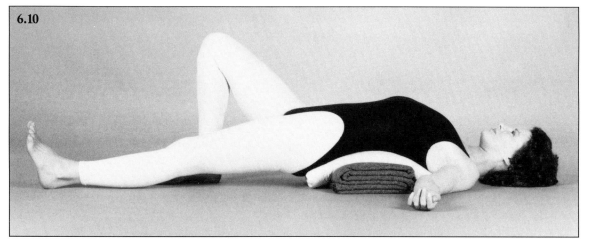

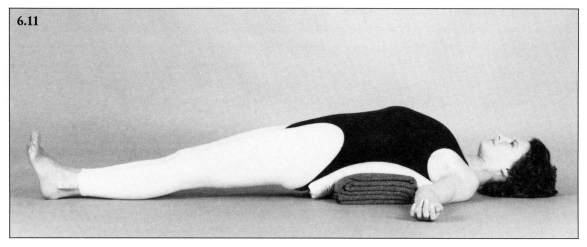

6.8   Passive Back Arch, Getting into Position
6.9   Passive Back Arch, Knees Bent
6.10   Passive Back Arch, One Leg Straight
6.11   Passive Back Arch, Legs Straight

To come out of the pose, on an exhalation, lift your right arm up until it points to the ceiling. Then roll over onto your back and notice how the stretch has made your body feel. Repeat on the other side. Do two to three sets.

Breathing and Imagery. While in the twist, visualize your spine lengthening and the muscles along the spine softening. Breathe quietly, using the Relaxation Breath and Total Torso Breathing.

Rationale. This relaxing passive spinal twist gently lengthens the paraspinals to increase the space between the vertebrae for proper disc nourishment and healing. It also stretches the pectoral muscles in the front of the chest, helping to correct rounded shoulders.

Note

• *Do not practice this pose during the second half of pregnancy.*

❈

Passive Back Arch

Props needed: two firm blankets

Position and Adustment. Fold each blanket in half lengthwise. Then fanfold them neatly so each one forms a pad four to eight inches thick and ten to twelve inches wide. (If you have a yoga bolster, it can be used instead. See Resources.) Place one blanket crosswise on top of the other.

Sit on the end of the top blanket, with your knees bent and your feet flat on the floor. It is important to use your arms for support as you gently let your torso down to lie on the blankets (Figure 6.8). Your shoulders and the back of your head should rest on the floor. Keep your knees bent as you begin to relax into the pose (Figure 6.9).

Then, on an exhalation, slide your left heel out on the floor until the leg is straight (Figure 6.10). See how that movement feels to your lower back. Inhale, and on the next exhalation, slide your left leg back to the starting position—knee bent, foot on the floor.

Inhale, and on the next exhalation, slide your right heel out until your leg is straight. Observe how that makes your lower back feel. Note any difference between the two sides. Return to both knees bent, feet on the floor.

Inhale and slowly slide your right heel out. If your lower back is comfortable, slowly slide your left heel out until both legs are extended (Figure 6.11). If your lower back is still comfortable, rest here for one to three minutes. If not, return to the bent-knees position. Lift your buttocks and lengthen the lower back by doing a pelvic tilt. Set your buttocks back down. Then try extending both legs again. If your lower back is still not comfortable, return to the bent-knees position (Figure 6.9), and rest there for one to three minutes.

If it is impossible to get comfortable even with both knees bent, try using blankets that are not so thick.

Breathing and Imagery. Use the Relaxation Breath. Imagine your spine as a smooth arch over the blankets. Visualize your spine as a gracefully arching bridge, effortlessly transferring your weight to its foundations on either side of a river.

Rationale. This pose provides gentle stretching of the pectoral (front chest) muscles, to relieve rounded shoulders. It stretches the muscles of the back of the neck, as well as the iliopsoas and quadriceps muscles, which bend the thigh at the hip and maintain the normal lumbar curve.

In those with a flat lumbar curve, this pose encourages a more normal curve. In those with a normal or increased curve, stretching of the chest and hip muscles reduces the excessive demands for movement placed on the lumbar spine by tight shoulders and hips. Also, lengthening the front thigh muscles and hip flexors (which attach to the pelvis and lumbar spine) keeps them from pulling the pelvis and lumbar spine into an exaggerated curve.

Note

• *Do not practice this pose during the second half of pregnancy.*

❧

Easy Bridge Pose

Props needed: neatly folded blanket.

Position and Adjustment, Variation 1. Lie on your back with your blanket under your shoulders, knees bent. Place your feet parallel, flat on the floor, with your heels close to your buttocks and hip-width apart. Have your thighs parallel and your arms at your sides, palms up.

On an exhalation, press your lower back into the floor by using the abdominal muscles to draw the pubic bone toward the breastbone, tilting the pelvis. Hold this position during the next inhalation. On the next exhalation, begin to lift your buttocks by pressing your feet firmly into the floor while maintaining a strong pelvic tilt. Lift your buttocks six to eight inches off the floor, keeping your breathing relaxed and your eyes looking down (Figure 6.12). Maintain a firm pressure of your shoulders and elbows against the floor. To keep your thighs from separating, press evenly into the bottoms of your feet. Resist the tendency for the weight to shift to the outer edge of the foot by pressing down with the inner heels. Keep your chest opening by moving your breastbone toward your head as much as you can. Your knees should stay hip-width apart. Keep your shoulders, jaw, and face relaxed.

Return to the starting position on an exhalation. As you lower your hips, keep the pubic bone moving toward the breastbone and the buttocks sweeping toward the backs of the knees. Repeat three to six times.

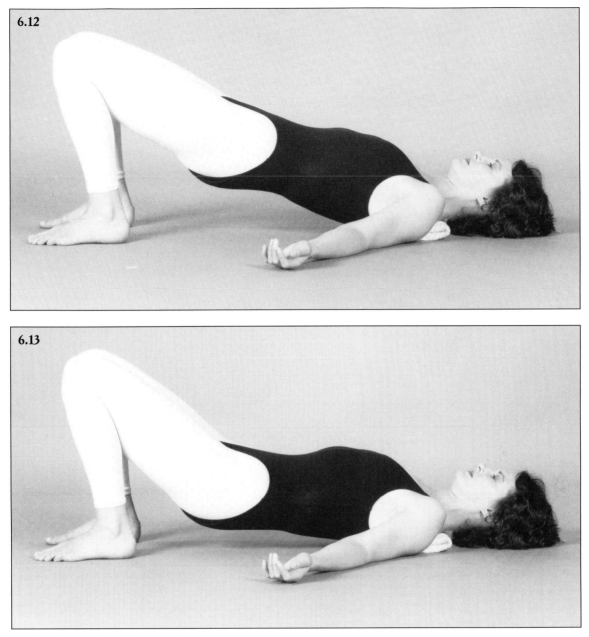

6.12

6.13

6.12   Easy Bridge Pose, Variation 1
6.13   Easy Bridge Pose, Variation 2

Variation 2. If you can't raise your buttocks six to eight inches, don't despair. Concentrate on drawing the pubic bone toward the breastbone and on pressing your feet firmly into the floor. From there, lift your buttocks any amount; even a half-inch will allow you to benefit from the pose (Figure 6.13).

Note

• *If you have spondylolysis or spondylolisthesis, do only Variation 2, lifting the buttocks no more than one to three inches from the floor.*

Breathing and Imagery. Breathe smoothly, quietly, and gently, coordinating the breath with the pose. Move only on an exhalation. Do not hold your breath.

Visualize your spine as a string of beads that is in a straight line when your lower back is pressed to the floor. Imagine lifting one bead at a time as you raise your buttocks and lower back. In returning to the starting position, replace the beads in the reverse order, with the one most recently lifted being the first to be returned to the floor.

Rationale. This pose strengthens the buttock muscles, the hamstrings, and the abdominals. It stretches the hip flexors, corrects both flat and increased lumbar curves, and improves rounded shoulders.

Note

• *Do not practice this pose during the second half of pregnancy.*

✤

One Leg Up, One Leg Out

Props needed: neck support roll, head pad.
(As needed: lumbar pad, rolled blanket.)

Position and Adjustment. Find a place, such as a doorway, where you can stretch one leg up the wall and stretch the other straight on the floor.

Sit with your right side close to the wall. Then, supporting your trunk with your arms, lie down and extend your right leg up the wall. Support your neck and head with your neck support roll and head pad. Keep your left leg bent, with the foot on the floor. Let your arms rest easily at your sides (Figure 6.14).

Adjust the position of your buttocks so that your right leg can be fully straightened and your sacrum can rest solidly on the floor. If you can't completely straighten your right leg, move your buttocks away from the wall until you can straighten your leg while maintaining a comfortable hamstring stretch. The feeling in the hamstrings should be muscle stretch, not overstretch pain.

Once the buttocks are positioned, slowly stretch out your left leg. If your lower back hurts when your left leg is outstretched on the floor, place a rolled blanket behind

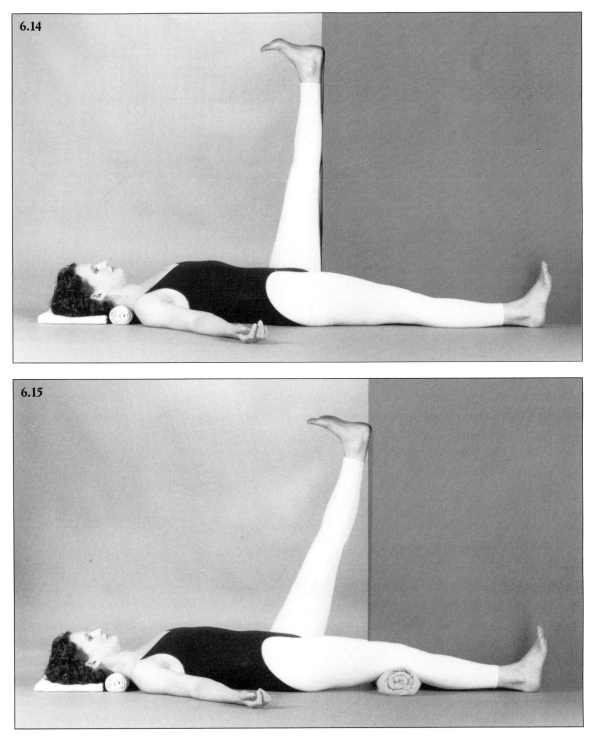

6.14 One Leg Up, One Leg Out
6.15 One Leg Up, One Leg Out, for Limited Flexibility

your knee so your lower back is comfortable (Figure 6.15). Repeat on the other side. Hold each side for two to five minutes.

For a greater challenge, bend the knee of the raised leg, and then actively straighten the leg as you pull back on the toes and stretch up through the heel. This will intensify the stretch, so go easy!

Breathing and Imagery. Use the Relaxation Breath. Visualize lengthening any muscles where you feel stretch.

Rationale. This position allows you to stretch the hamstrings of one leg and the hip flexors of the other leg.

Notes

- *If you have a flat back, use your lumbar pad.*
- *If this pose aggravates your sciatica, try moving the buttocks farther from the wall. If that does not eliminate the pain, delete it for now and work on the standing poses in the next chapter ("Moving On Poses") for a month before trying it again.*
- *If you have scoliosis, spondylolysis, or spondylolisthesis, this pose is important for you.*
- *Do not practice this pose during the second half of pregnancy.*
- *If you notice an asymmetry in hamstring flexibility, you may also have pelvic torsion, caused by uneven pulling of the hamstrings on the pelvis. See Chapter 8, "Sacroiliac Pain and Sciatica."*

❧

Kneeling Lunge

Props needed: chair, mat or blanket
for kneeling comfort.

Position, Adjustment, Breathing, and Imagery. Kneel in front of a chair. Place your left foot in front of you so that your knee is at a ninety-degree angle directly over your ankle. Hold the chair for balance, if necessary. Keep your torso erect and your ears over your shoulders (Figure 6.16).

Inhale into your entire torso. As you exhale, lift your pubic bone toward your breastbone and tuck your tailbone, so you feel a stretch across the front of your right groin and down the front of your right thigh (Figure 6.17). (This is the same pelvic movement as in Supine Pelvic Tilt, Figure 6.1.) Keep your breastbone lifting to avoid collapsing your chest. Don't lean forward into the lunge (Figure 6.18, Incorrect); keep your knee directly over your ankle. Hold the stretch for several breaths, allowing your front thigh muscles to soften and lengthen.

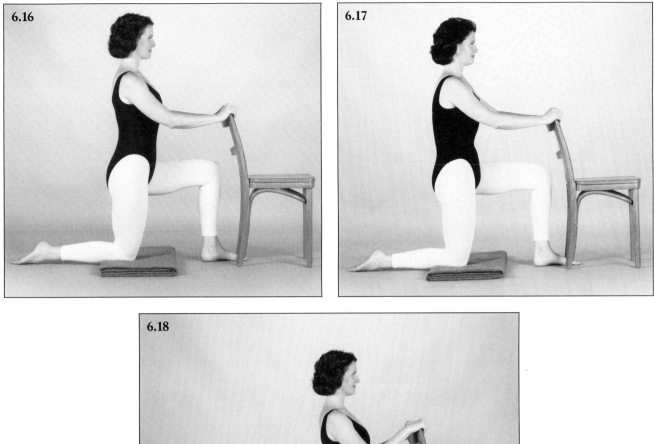

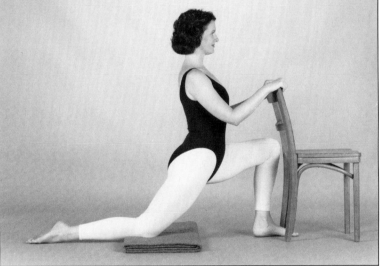

6.16   Kneeling Lunge, Starting Position
6.17   Kneeling Lunge, with Pubic Bone Lifted
6.18   Kneeling Lunge, Incorrect

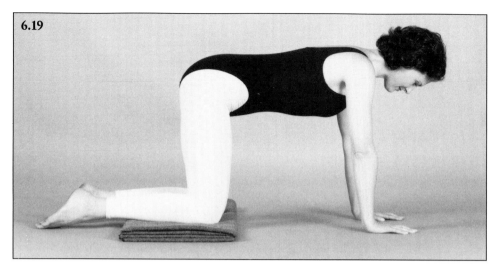

6.19

6.20

6.21

6.19 **All Fours, Starting Position**
6.20 **All Fours, Variation 1**
6.21 **All Fours, Variation 2**

Repeat with the right foot in front, feeling the stretch in the left thigh and groin. Do three to five sets.

Rationale. This pose stretches the hip flexors (which attach to the front of the lumbar vertebrae and the back top rim of the pelvis), thus decreasing their forward pull on the lumbar vertebrae. It is also an abdominal strengthener. Abdominal strengthening and hip flexor stretching are important to those with a normal or increased lumbar curve.

Notes

- *If you have a flat back, practice this exercise with the arms raised overhead to encourage a more normal lumbar arch.*
- *If you have spondylolysis or spondylolisthesis, this pose is important to master, as it reduces the tendency of tight hip flexors to pull the lumbar spine forward over the sacrum.*
- *This pose can be used throughout pregnancy for release of lower back tension. Don't raise the arms overhead.*

✢

All Fours

Prop needed: knee pad.

Position and Adjustment. Kneel on all fours, with your knees directly under your hips and your hands directly under your shoulders (Figure 6.19). Use a pad under your knees for comfort. Do not raise your head; rather, keep your head and chin in the same relationship to your neck and shoulders as they would be in if you were standing. Also keep your lower back in neutral alignment, neither flattened or overarched. (To check your lower back alignment, first round it, then overarch it; then find the correct position, half-way in between.)

Variation 1. On an exhalation, raise one arm, stretch it forward, hold it for several breaths (Figure 6.20), and then lower it. Keep your shoulders moving away from your ears. To prevent your lower back from overarching, keep your lower front ribs moving into your body, your pubic bone moving toward your navel, and your buttocks sweeping toward the backs of your knees. If you can't keep your back from overarching, lower your arm. If lifting the arm straight ahead irritates the shoulder joint, try lifting it out to the side. If the shoulders become sore, decrease the duration and number of repetitions and build up more gradually. Repeat on the other side.

Variation 2. On an exhalation, straighten one leg, and then raise it without allowing your lower back to overarch (Figure 6.21). Keep the raised leg active by stretching out through the heel. Hold the leg up for several breaths and then lower it. If lifting the out-stretched leg causes back pain, keep the knee bent and lift the knee only a few inches off the floor. Repeat on the other side.

Do several sets of Variations 1 and 2. As strength improves over the months, gradually increase the length of time you hold the pose and the number of repetitions.

Breathing and Imagery. Keep your breath flowing smoothly, without restriction. Do not hold your breath. Feel how the muscles of your spine are activated as you lift your limbs. See your paraspinal muscles getting stronger.

Rationale. Lifting the arms or legs strengthens the paraspinal muscles on either side of the spine. The buttock muscles are strengthened, providing better pelvic support and greater leg strength for proper lifting. Also strengthened are the muscles that stabilize the shoulder blades and help counter rounded shoulders. The pose also teaches awareness and control of the lumbar curve.

Notes

- *If you have spondylolysis or spondylolisthesis, make sure you are not exaggerating your lumbar curve. (Use a mirror or have a helper check to see if you are swaybacked in the pose.)*
- *If you can't control your lumbar curve, delete this pose for now and work on the preceding poses that strengthen the abdominals and help you maintain good lumbar and pelvic alignment. Try the pose again after a few months.*

❧

Mountain Pose

Props needed: nonskid surface or mat

Position and Adjustment. Stand with bare feet parallel to each other. Place your feet three to five inches apart, directly under the hips (Figure 6.22). Spread your toes so you can see space between them. If your big toes point toward the outside of your foot instead of straight ahead, bend your knees to reach down and move them over toward the midline, so that they are more properly aligned. Do this every time you practice Mountain Pose, even though they may not stay where you put them at first.

While standing erect, become aware of the weight distribution on the bottoms of your feet. Is there more weight on one foot than the other? Is there more weight on the heel or the ball of each foot? The weight should be equal on the two feet and distributed evenly between the heels and the balls of the feet.

If your toes are trying to grip the floor, relax them. If they seem to be stuck in a claw or hammer shape, practice lifting them off the floor.

If you have flat feet, shift your weight slightly toward the little toe side of the foot to create more of an arch. In doing so, don't allow the base of the big toe to leave the floor.

If you have high arches, make sure that you are pressing down as strongly with the base of the big toe and the inner aspect of the heel as you are with the outer side of the foot.

Activating the Legs. Learning to activate the muscles above and below the knee is a vital step in gaining the leg and buttock strength and stability needed to support your back in daily activities and exercise. This same action is used in the other standing yoga poses to create strength and stability. Activating the legs helps correct several types of knee misalignments, such as hyperextension, knock knees, and functional bowlegs.

To activate your legs, stand so that the center lines of your feet (imaginary lines drawn from between the second and third toes to each heel) are parallel. While keeping your upper body erect (keep lengthening up from the center of the top of the head), bend your knees so that they move out over the center lines of the feet (Figure 6.23). Don't allow the knees to come together or splay apart. Don't allow the lumbar curve to increase.

Inhale, and on the next exhalation, slowly begin to straighten your legs by pushing your feet into the floor while straightening your knees. Again, don't let your knees come together or separate, but keep them moving parallel to each other. Imagine someone is pressing into the backs of your knees trying to keep you from straightening them. Do not allow the knees to go past straight to a hyperextended position—be sure to stop the backward motion of the knee joint at a normal straight-leg position. (It may be helpful to have a friend or a mirror nearby to tell you about the exact position of your knees. For most people who have habitual hyperextended knee posture, the normal straight-leg position will feel as though the knees are bent.)

Be aware of the feeling of the muscles working in your calves and thighs as the legs are straightened. *Once the straight-leg position is attained, maintain this muscle activity,* keeping the leg muscles working, for thirty to sixty seconds. During this time, return your awareness to balance and alignment, focusing on evenly distributing the weight on the bottoms of the feet and on lengthening up from the center of the top of your head without raising your chin. Note that each leg is active and straight, but *the knees are not locked.* Practice this standing posture often during the day as well as during your exercise period.

Breathing and Imagery. Feel the pull of gravity on your feet and visualize your connection to the Earth. Imagine yourself as a mountain with a broad solid base topped by a lofty peak that reaches into the clouds. Imagine yourself as a strong, tall tree with deep roots and a crown of leafy branches reaching for the sun. Allow yourself to feel taller than you think you are.

Breath smoothly and easily. With each inhalation feel your mountain or tree growing taller. With each exhalation enjoy your new height.

Rationale. This deceptively simple standing pose is the basis for back rehabilitation through yoga. It provides the lessons of postural awareness, pelvic positioning, and leg strengthening that are crucial to back health. You will carry lessons of balance and alignment from this posture into the more complicated and challenging standing poses (described in Chapter 7), which help develop back, leg, and abdominal strength for back support.

Mountain Pose and the other standing poses also send body language messages of inner strength, being able to stand on your own two feet, and doing something positive for yourself.

✣

Standing Twist

Prop needed: sturdy chair, nonskid surface.

Position and Adjustment. Place a sturdy chair on a nonskid surface next to a kitchen counter, banister rail, or wall. Stand in front of the chair with your left side next to the wall. Begin by performing Mountain Pose with activated legs, balancing evenly on your feet and visualizing the center point of the top of your head moving toward the ceiling. Then gradually shift your weight to your right foot and place your left foot on the chair seat, so that the left knee is bent at about ninety degrees (Figure 6.24). Recheck your lumbar curve, making sure that it is neither increased nor decreased in this position.

Inhale, and on the exhalation, gradually begin twisting your torso toward the wall. As you twist, keep lengthening up from the top of your head. Keep your right leg activated. Do not allow your chest to slump. Keep the muscles of your jaw and neck relaxed and your chin level. The movement should originate from the base of the spinal column and the abdomen. Let your head and neck move as a consequence of twisting the torso, rather than twisting the head and neck first and moving the torso secondarily.

Coordinate the twist and the upward movement with the breath in the following way: On one inhalation and exhalation, stand still, focusing on a strong connection of your feet with the floor and chair seat and on lifting up from the top of your head. With the next inhalation, soften your neck and jaw muscles, and on the exhalation, increase the twist slightly. Continue in this manner, *increasing the twist only on every alternate exhalation.* Never twist aggressively.

When you've attained your maximum twist, place your hands on the wall or counter for stability (Figure 6.25). Stay there for several breaths before slowly and gently releasing the twist. Allow yourself to become tall as you untwist. Compare the feelings on the right and left sides of your spine. Repeat on the other side. Do three to six sets.

Breathing and Imagery. Breathing should be gentle and carefully coordinated with the twist. Imagine your spine as a coiled spring that is released on every exhalation to either lengthen upward or to rotate about its axis.

Rationale. This pose strengthens and stretches the spinal rotators and abdominal muscles, as well as strengthening the legs, buttocks, and upper back.

Notes

- *If you feel little or no stretch in your straight leg or in the buttock of the bent leg, try using a chair or stool that is several inches higher.*
- *Do not practice this pose during the second half of pregnancy.*

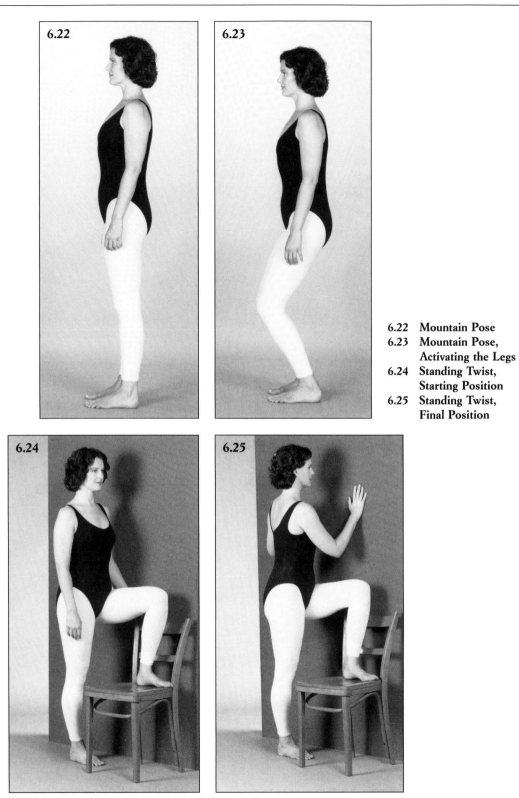

6.22　Mountain Pose
6.23　Mountain Pose,
　　　Activating the Legs
6.24　Standing Twist,
　　　Starting Position
6.25　Standing Twist,
　　　Final Position

• *If you have spondylolysis or spondylolisthesis, this is another important pose for you. Before you twist, make sure that your back is not overarched.*

Suggested Routines

Ten Minutes

1. Supine Pelvic Tilt, four sets (Figure 6.1)
2. Yoga Sit-Ups, four sets (Figures 6.2–6.4)
3. Mountain Pose, activating the legs, one minute (Figures 6.22, 6.23)
4. Kneeling Lunge, two sets (Figures 6.16, 6.17)
5. Crocodile Twist, two sets (Figure 6.7)
6. Supine Child's Pose, one minute (Figure 5.10)
7. Child's Pose, remaining time (Figure 5.11)

Twenty Minutes

1. Yoga Sit-Ups, four sets (Figures 6.2–6.4)
2. One Leg Up, One Leg Out, two minutes each side (Figure 6.14)
3. Mountain Pose, activating the legs, one minute (Figures 6.22, 6.23)
4. Kneeling Lunge, two sets, two minutes (Figures 6.16, 6.17)
5. Supine Knee-Chest Twist, Variation 1, thirty seconds each side (Figure 6.5)
6. Supine Knee-Chest Twist, Variation 2, three sets (Figure 6.6)
7. Standing Twist, two sets (Figures 6.24, 6.25)
8. Passive Back Arch, one minute (Figures 6.8–6.11)
9. Easy Bridge Pose, two times (Figures 6.12, 6.13)
10. All Fours, Variation 1, two sets (Figure 6.20)
11. All Fours, Variation 2, two sets (Figure 6.21)
12. Supine Child's Pose, two minutes (Figure 5.10)
13. Lying Down with Calves on a Chair, two minutes (Figure 5.7)

Thirty Minutes

1. Supine Pelvic Tilt, four times (Figure 6.1)
2. Yoga Sit-Ups, four sets (Figures 6.2–6.4)
3. One Leg Up, One Leg Out, two minutes each side (Figure 6.14)
4. Mountain Pose, activating the legs, one minute (Figures 6.22, 6.23)
5. Kneeling Lunge, two sets (Figures 6.16, 6.17)
6. Supine Knee-Chest Twist, Variation 1, two sets (Figure 6.5)
7. Supine Knee-Chest Twist, Variation 2, two sets (Figure 6.6)
8. Crocodile Twist, two sets (Figure 6.7)
9. Standing Twist, three sets (Figures 6.24, 6.25)
10. Passive Back Arch, one minute (Figures 6.8–6.11)
11. Easy Bridge Pose, three times (Figure 6.12, 6.13)
12. All Fours, Variation 1, two sets (Figure 6.20)
13. All Fours, Variation 2, two sets (Figure 6.21)
14. Supine Child's Pose, one minute (Figure 5.10)
15. Child's Pose, one minute (Figure 5.11)
16. Lying Down with Calves on a Chair, remaining time (Figure 5.7)

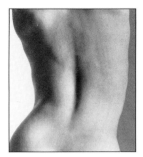

Seven

Moving on Poses

*O*nce you are familiar with the Home Base poses and can do them without pain, you can begin to gradually add Moving On poses. These slightly more challenging poses continue the process of recovery by building on the strength, flexibility, and postural correction skills fostered in the previous chapters.

Add only one new pose every two or three weeks, so you have time to evaluate the effects and demands of each additional pose. If back pain recurs after several new poses are added at once, it's hard to know which one caused the problem. But if just one new pose has been added, it will be clear where you need to direct more attention and awareness.

Each pose helps develop muscular strength and flexibility so habitual posture can improve. All the major posture-determining muscle groups are strengthened and any asymmetries are balanced out. Neuromuscular coordination is encouraged and reinforced.

All these factors combine to make lifting and getting up and down safer and to lessen the likelihood of falling and the risk of injury. Your sense of power and self-determination will increase with practice, as the postures send messages of strength, stability, and worthiness to your inner self.

Note

- *All the standing poses presented in this chapter can be performed throughout pregnancy as long as they are comfortable for you. The strength, endurance, and flexibility they develop ease the demands of childbirth and child care. In later months of pregnancy, you may wish to decrease the number of repetitions or the durations.*

Foot Tips for the Standing Poses

The careful placement of the feet and activation of the leg muscles in the standing poses offers an excellent opportunity for correcting foot and knee misalignment. Before beginning, practice basic standing awareness. Standing with your feet parallel, see if you can center your weight so that it is neither on the right foot nor the left foot, neither forward on the toes nor back on the heels, but centered equally just in front of the ankle on each foot.

If your toe knuckles are white when you practice the standing poses or if your toes are stuck in a claw or hammer shape, you must continuously tell them to let go. Distributing the weight evenly on the sole of the foot makes it easier not to grip with the toes. If you can't relax your toes, try to lift them off the floor without lifting the ball of the foot.

While practicing the standing poses, make sure the muscles of your legs are properly activated so your knees are straight but not locked. To remind yourself how to activate the legs, practice Mountain Pose (Chapter 6).

For Flat Feet. If your feet tend to be flat, resist this tendency by actively lifting the inner ankle bones, so your weight shifts more to the outside of your feet. As you do this, don't allow the base of your big toe to leave the floor. Notice that when you allow your feet to collapse into their habitual flat-footed position, your knees point inward. Notice, too, that when your feet are properly aligned, your knees also assume a more balanced alignment.

For High Arches. If your feet have high arches, and you tend to bear most of your weight on the outsides of your feet, resist this tendency. Press firmly down through your heels and the base of each big toe. Notice how this action affects knee alignment: Instead of pointing outward, the knees come into a more stable alignment facing forward directly over the center of the feet.

❈

Triangle Pose

Props needed: sturdy table, railing, or kitchen
counter; nonskid surface.

Position and Adjustment. Begin practicing this pose with a sturdy table, stable railing, or kitchen counter for support. Make sure the table won't slip when you lean against it. Use a noncarpeted floor or nonskid yoga mat to avoid slipping and to give yourself a firm base.

Stand in Mountain Pose (Figure 6.22) with your back to the table. Activate your legs. Step your feet apart about three and one-half to four feet, keeping them parallel (Figure 7.1). Breathe normally as you turn your left foot in and your right foot out, so the right foot is at a ninety-degree angle and the left foot at a fifteen-degree angle to the original starting position. The toes of both feet should point to the right and the right heel should

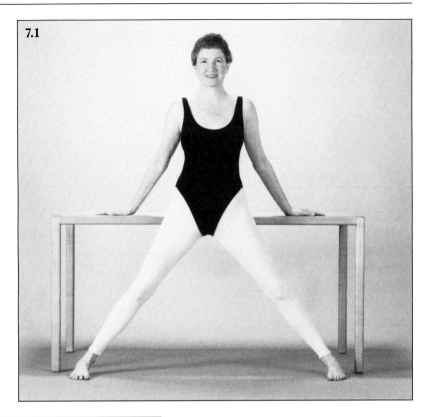

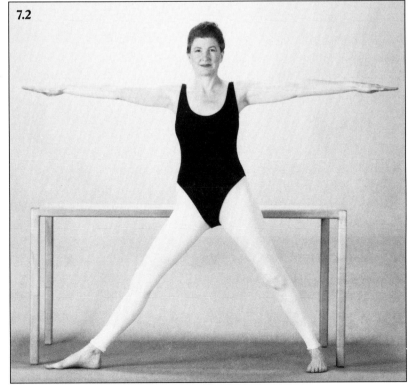

7.1 **Triangle Pose, Preparatory Stance**
7.2 **Triangle Pose, Feet in Position**

be directly in line with the center of the left arch. If you need support, hold the table; otherwise spread your arms and stretch out through your fingertips (Figure 7.2).

Inhaling, activate your legs again by pressing your heels into the floor. Exhaling, lengthen your spine upward, allowing yourself to be as tall as you can without lifting your chin or your shoulders. Inhale, and on an exhalation, bend to the right from the hip joint, so your torso bends sideways as a unit toward your right leg. Don't bend from your waist (Figure 7.3, Incorrect). Keep breathing normally. Rest your right hand or forearm on the table to provide support for your back and torso. Let your left hand rest on your left hip. Maintain the pose for one to three breaths, keeping your legs active and your neck and shoulders relaxed (Figure 7.4).

On an inhalation, come out of the pose by pressing into the floor with both feet and into the table with your right hand or forearm. Reach for the ceiling with your left hand, using this reaching action to lift your torso upright (Figure 7.5). Then turn your feet to face forward. Pause for a moment to feel the effects of the pose.

Repeat the sequence on the other side.

Do one to three sets of Triangle Pose for the first few months, gradually building up to six sets over six to eight months. As you become stronger in the pose, gradually rest less and less of your weight on the table (Figure 7.6).

Breathing and Imagery. Breathe with your entire torso. Experience strength and stability in the legs. Imagine that your feet are sending roots toward the center of the Earth, firmly anchoring you in the pose. Imagine that your spine is elongating with each breath, like a tree branch growing up and out.

Rationale. Triangle Pose strengthens all of the stabilizing muscles of the feet, legs, hips, and spine, especially the paraspinal and the abdominal muscles. If the paraspinals or the hamstrings are tight on one side of the body, Triangle Pose can help even out these differences by gradually lengthening the shorter side.

Note

- *If you experience pain or difficulty in Triangle Pose, try Revolved Triangle Pose (Figure 7.10) and Extended Warrior Pose (Figure 7.23). One of those may be much easier for you. If so, work on it for a few months before attempting Triangle Pose again.*

❀

Revolved Triangle Pose

Props needed: sturdy table, railing, or kitchen
counter; nonskid mat.

Position and Adjustment. The beginning leg position is the same as for Triangle Pose, already described. Stand in Mountain Pose with your back to the table, legs

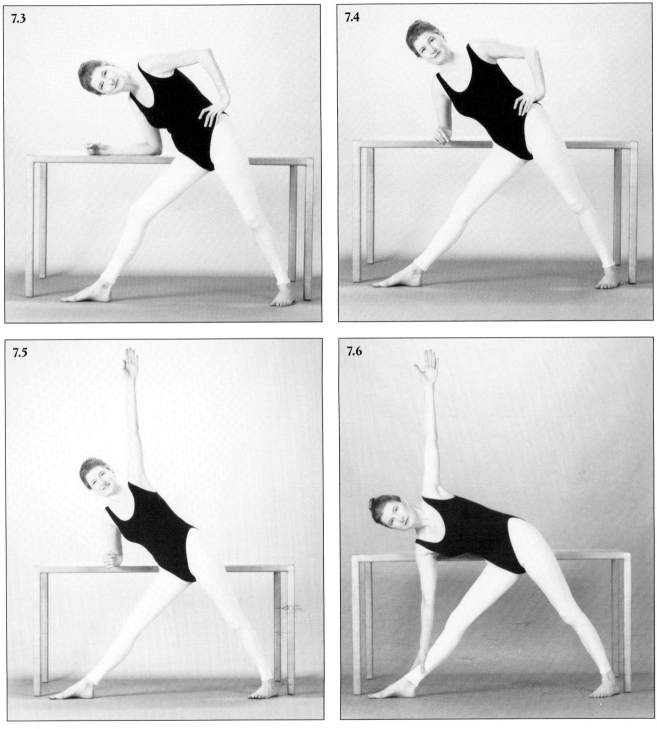

7.3   **Triangle Pose, Incorrect**
7.4   **Triangle Pose, Final Position with Table Support**
7.5   **Triangle Pose, Exiting the Pose**
7.6   **Triangle Pose, Final Position without Support**

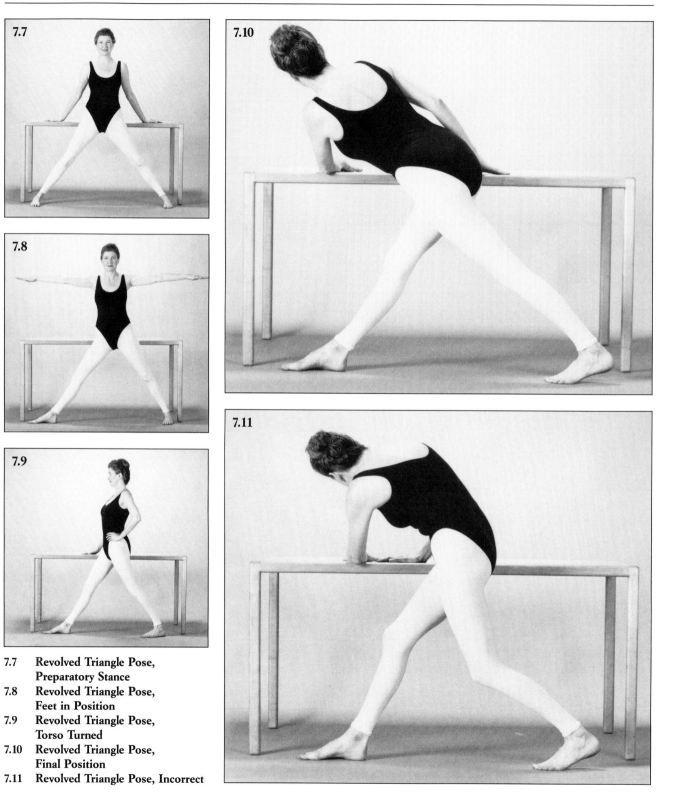

7.7   **Revolved Triangle Pose,
Preparatory Stance**
7.8   **Revolved Triangle Pose,
Feet in Position**
7.9   **Revolved Triangle Pose,
Torso Turned**
7.10   **Revolved Triangle Pose,
Final Position**
7.11   **Revolved Triangle Pose, Incorrect**

activated. On an inhalation, step your feet to a parallel position three and one-half to four feet apart (Figure 7.7). Exhale and activate your legs. Inhaling, spread your arms out to the sides. While exhaling, turn your left foot in and your right foot out, with your right heel in line with your left arch (Figure 7.8). Keep your legs activated by continuously pressing your heels into the floor.

Inhale, and on the exhalation, turn your hips so the front of your torso points in the same direction as your right leg (Figure 7.9). Inhale and lengthen your spine. While exhaling, bend forward from your hips (not your waist), using both hands on the table for support. Keep rotating your trunk to face the table, twisting the torso as a unit about the axis of the spine (Figure 7.10). Feel your abdomen sweep from the left to the right as the torso continues to lengthen. Your left heel will probably come off the floor—that's okay. Don't distort the spinal alignment by bending at your waist or allowing your back to round (Figure 7.11, Incorrect).

Stay in this position for one to three breaths, pressing your feet into the floor and lengthening your spine. Keep your jaw relaxed and your breathing quiet and easy.

On an inhalation, come out of the pose by pressing down with both arms and both legs. Pause to feel the effects of the pose. Then repeat it on the other side.

At first, practice this pose for one to three sets, holding for one to three breaths. Over six to eight months, gradually increase the number of repetitions to six sets. As you become stronger in the pose, rest less and less of your weight on the table.

Breathing and Imagery. Visualize roots holding each foot firmly to the floor. See how the firm base formed by your feet and legs allows your spine to lengthen as you practice Total Torso Breathing. Let a feeling of weightlessness permeate your torso with each breath. Breathing out, release all heaviness and stiffness.

Rationale. The stretching, strengthening, stabilizing, and balancing effects of this pose are similar to those described for Triangle Pose. Working in the revolved position provides additional stretching and strengthening for the small rotator muscles of the spine and the outer muscles of the hips and thighs.

✻

Half-Moon Pose

Props needed: sturdy table, stable railing, or kitchen
counter; nonskid surface.

Position and Adjustment. This balancing position begins with Triangle Pose. Stand in Mountain Pose, with your back to a sturdy table, stable railing, or kitchen counter. Activate your legs by pressing the heels firmly down. While inhaling, step your feet three and one-half to four feet apart. While exhaling, turn your feet to the right to assume the basic Triangle Pose stance, resting your right hand or forearm on the table for support.

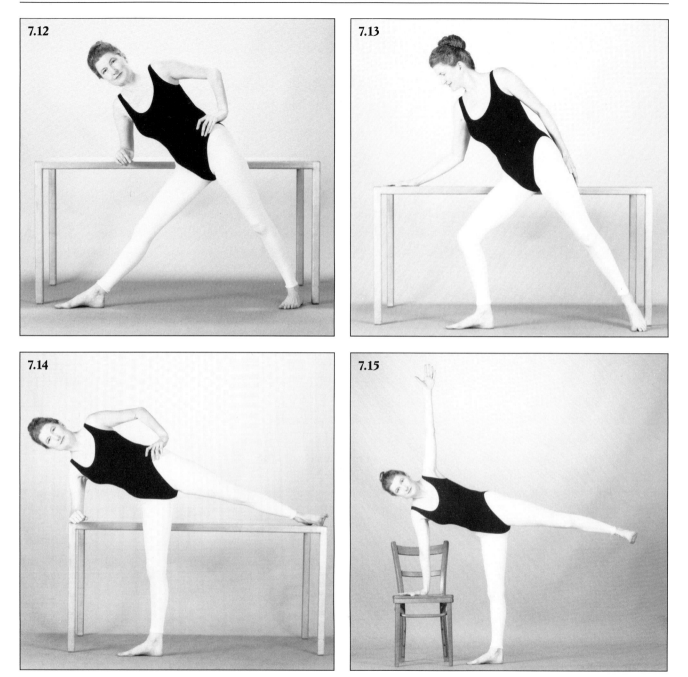

7.12   Half Moon Pose, Preparation
7.13   Half Moon Pose, Transition from Triangle Pose
7.14   Half Moon Pose, Final Position with Table
7.15   Half Moon Pose, Final Position with Chair

Inhale and reactivate the legs. While exhaling, bend at the hip to assume Triangle Pose (Figure 7.12). Pause to enjoy it.

Inhale. On the exhalation, bend your right knee as you shift your weight onto your right foot (Figure 7.13). Lift the left leg so that it is parallel to the floor while straightening the right leg. Keep both knees straight and both legs firm. Use the support of the table for stability. Let your left arm rest on the left side of your body. If you are flexible enough, let the outstretched left leg rest on the table (Figure 7.14). Otherwise, lift it just as high as you can.

To keep your spine properly aligned and your torso straight throughout the entire process, keep lengthening the lower side of the torso from the right hip to the armpit. Don't forget to breathe. Hold the pose for one to three breaths, breathing gently and feeling a solid connection of the right foot with the floor and a strong extension through the left heel.

Stay in the balanced position only as long as you remain stable and able to come out of the pose with control. Make sure that both knees and both legs remain straight and activated once balance is achieved.

There are two ways to come out of the pose: Place the left leg on the floor and return to Mountain Pose, or return to Triangle Pose and then stand up. After coming out of the pose, pause to feel its effects. Repeat on the other side.

Do one to three sets for the first several months. Over six to eight months, gradually increase to six sets. Once you can comfortably perform five to six sets, begin to use a lower support such as a chair seat (Figure 7.15). As you progress, rely on the table less for support, using it only for balance.

Breathing and Imagery. Use Total Torso Breathing. With each inhalation, visualize strong roots extending down from the soles of your feet to anchor you solidly to the floor. With each exhalation, feel your spine and your raised leg floating light and long. Elongate from the tips of your toes to the top of your head.

Rationale. In addition to the benefits of Triangle Pose, Half-Moon Pose exercises the muscles that support the foot arch, knee, hip joint, and spine. It stretches the hamstrings and inner thigh muscles and strengthens all of the main movers and supporters of the legs, hips, spine, and shoulder girdle. This pose also helps even out any asymmetries on the two sides of the body, by stretching tight muscles and strengthening weak ones.

🍃

Warrior Pose

Props needed: sturdy table or kitchen counter;
nonskid surface.

Position and Adjustment. Start in Mountain Pose, with your back to a sturdy table or kitchen counter. Activate your legs by pressing your heels firmly into the floor.

While inhaling, step your feet four to five feet apart, depending on your height and flexibility (Figure 7.16). If you are short or inflexible, your legs will not be as wide apart as if you are tall or very flexible. Let the width of the stance be dictated by your feeling of stability and balance in the pose. You should feel some stretch in the legs, but no pain.

Exhale, keeping your legs active and straight. While inhaling, turn your left foot in and your right foot out, as in Triangle Pose (Figure 7.17). While exhaling, bend your right knee until the knee is exactly over the ankle (Figure 7.18). If the knee is beyond the ankle and over the foot, the stance should be wider (Figure 7.19, Incorrect). If the knee will not reach to a position over the ankle, the stance is too wide (Figure 7.20, Incorrect). If the knee tends to move toward the big-toe side of your foot, gently return it to its proper position exactly over the ankle.

If necessary, press your arms and hands against the table behind you for support. Hold the pose, keeping your left leg straight and activated, for one to three breaths.

Carefully observe the alignment of both feet. Feel the weight evenly distributed over the base of each foot. If you tend toward flat feet, do not allow the arches to collapse inward. If you tend toward high arches, resist the urge to shift the weight to the little toe side of the foot.

Remember to keep your spine aligned in its normal spinal curves. Allow the spine to lengthen upward. Relax your shoulders and jaw and remember to breathe.

On an inhalation, come out of the pose with control by pressing firmly down with your right foot as you straighten the leg. Pause to feel the effects of the pose, breathing quietly. Turn your feet in the opposite direction, and repeat the pose on the left side.

Start with one to three sets of the pose for the first few months of practice. Then, during the next six to eight months, gradually build up to six sets. Once you are doing five to six sets, begin practicing one to two of them with your back close to a wall instead of the table (for support in case you need it). Gradually decrease your use of the table (Figure 7.21).

Breathing and Imagery. Keep your breathing smooth and easy while practicing Warrior Pose. The usual tendency is to breathe rapidly or hold your breath, either of which makes the pose much more difficult. With each Total Torso inhalation, visualize long, strong roots growing from the soles of your feet toward the center of the Earth. With each exhalation, release your heaviness and fatigue. As your roots grow down, feel your spine grow upward.

Rationale. This vigorous standing pose continues the work of the preceding postures to increase strength in the spine-supporting muscles of the legs, buttocks, back, and abdomen. It teaches coordinated, properly aligned movements and stretches the muscles of the legs, pelvic girdle, and buttocks.

The body language of Warrior Pose reflects its name: It speaks of solid self-sufficiency, self-confidence, and inner strength.

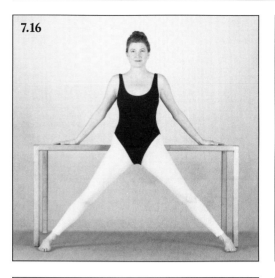

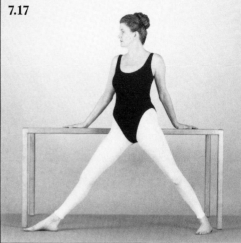

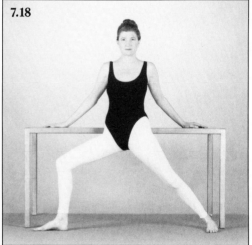

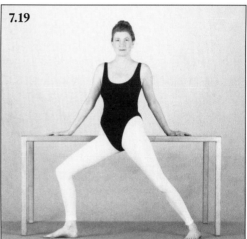

7.16 Warrior Pose,
    Preparatory Stance
7.17 Warrior Pose, Feet
    in Position
7.18 Warrior Pose,
    Final Position
    with Support
7.19 Warrior Pose,
    Incorrect, Stance
    Too Narrow
7.20 Warrior Pose,
    Incorrect, Stance
    Too Wide
7.21 Warrior Pose,
    Final Position
    without Support

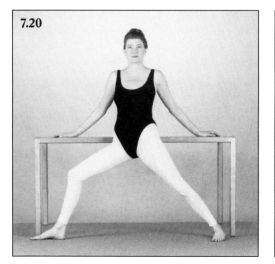

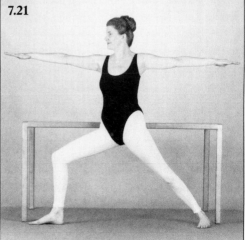

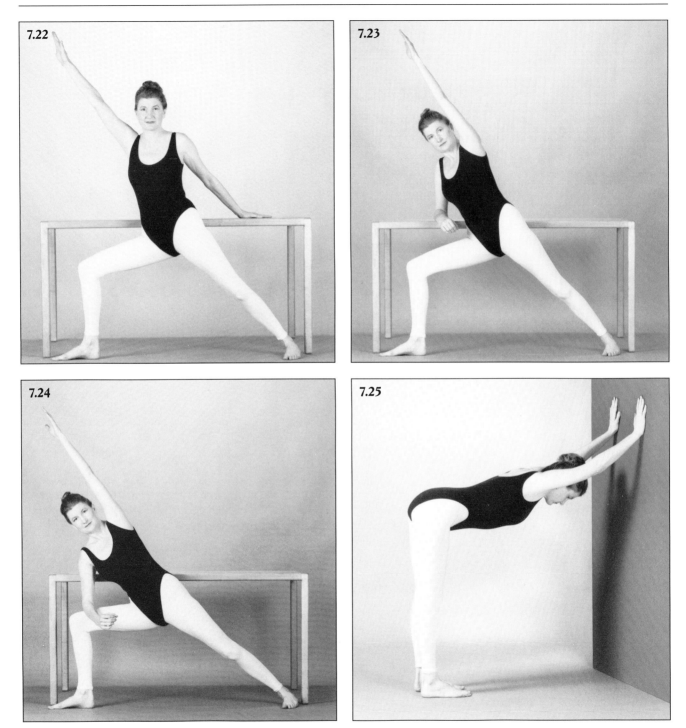

7.22 Extended Warrior Pose, Going into the Pose
7.23 Extended Warrior Pose, Final Position with Support
7.24 Extended Warrior Pose, Final Position without Support
7.25 Wall Push

❧ Extended Warrior Pose

Props needed: sturdy table, nonskid surface.

Position and Adjustment. Start in Warrior Pose with the right knee bent. While breathing naturally, stretch your right arm up toward the ceiling, reaching out with your fingers (Figure 7.22). Keeping the right side of your body long, tilt your entire trunk so your right forearm can rest on the table (Figure 7.23) or your thigh (Figure 7.24). Be sure to bend from the right hip, not from the waist. (If you have to bend at your waist to put your elbow on your thigh, rest it on the table instead.) Keep your legs active by firmly pushing your heels into the floor. Once you are steady, reach your left arm across your left ear so it forms a continuous line with your left leg.

If your back is especially sore, try elevating the ball of the foot (on the bent-leg side) on a book or block of wood two to three inches thick.

Stay in the pose for one to three breaths, breathing easily, eyes open and looking down. Repeat on the other side.

Breathing and Imagery. In your mind's eye, see a straight line extending from the sole of your back foot to the fingertips of your raised hand. Let that line elongate with each exhalation.

Rationale. This pose builds upon the work of the other standing poses to provide strength, coordination, and flexibility to the supporting structures of the back. If you have difficulty with Triangle Pose, you might find this pose much easier. Practice this pose instead of Triangle Pose for several months before trying Triangle Pose again.

❧ Wall Push

Props needed: nonskid surface, wall.

Position and Adjustment. Stand facing a bare wall, about a foot away from it, feet parallel and six to eight inches apart. Place your hands on the wall at shoulder height, shoulder-width apart, with your middle fingers parallel and pointing at the ceiling. Stand in Mountain Pose with your legs activated.

While inhaling and pushing your hands into the wall, step back as you bend forward from the hips (not the waist). Keep your torso aligned in its normal spinal curves (Figure 7.25). If this position gives you too much stretch in the backs of your thighs or pain in your lower back, step forward toward the wall and reposition your hands a little higher, at the level of your face. Then step back and bend forward from your hips again, assessing the amount of stretch in your hamstrings. If the stretch is tolerable, this may be your proper position. If it is not tolerable, try it with your hands even higher, until you reach a position

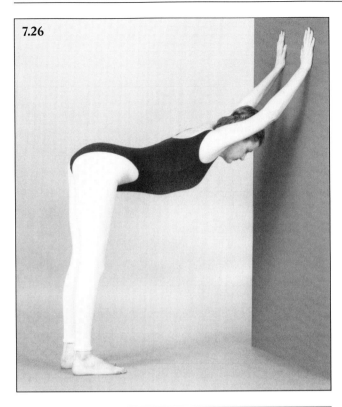

7.26

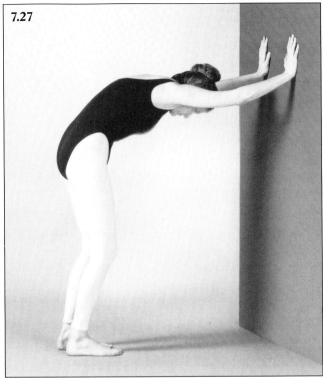

7.27

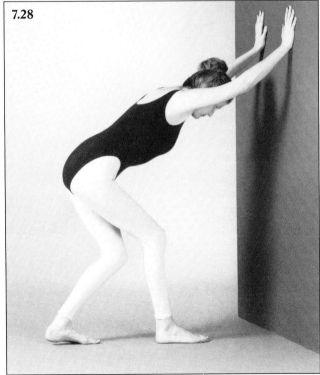

7.28

7.26 Wall Push, Incorrect, Lumbar Overarched
7.27 Wall Push, Incorrect, Hands Too Low for Limited Flexibility
7.28 Wall Push, Step Forward to Exit Pose

where you feel a comfortable stretch in the hamstrings while bending forward at the hips and retaining the normal alignment of your spine.

Your spine and torso should have the same configuration that they do when you are in your normal standing posture: Your lower back should not be either overarched (Figure 7.26, Incorrect) or rounded (Figure 7.27, Incorrect), and your upper back should not be rounded any more than it usually is. The key to proper spinal alignment in this pose is bending from your hips rather than from your waist. If you don't have a large mirror available to let you see the alignment of your back, a helper can provide this information.

If you feel discomfort in your shoulders, place your hands wider apart. Do not allow your elbows to hyperextend (that is, to go past straight). If they do, bend them slightly until they are straight and then hold them in that position by actively pushing your hands into the wall.

Stay in the pose for one to three breaths, breathing easily. Keep your legs active by firmly pressing your heels into the floor. To come out of the pose, bend your knees slightly and step forward toward the wall, so that you bring your legs under your body before standing (Figure 7.28). Stand quietly to let the effects of the pose sink into your awareness.

Repeat two to three times.

Breathing and Imagery. With every inhalation, imagine roots extending down into the floor from your feet and into the wall from your hands. Visualize your spine growing longer so that the top of your head moves toward the wall. See rounded shoulders melting away as your chest opens. Breathe softness into your ribs and length into your hamstring muscles. Breathe serenely and effortlessly. Keep your jaw relaxed.

Rationale. Excellent for removing fatigue and releasing tight, tired back muscles, Wall Push is a great all-purpose pose that works well for all types of bodies, both flexible and stiff. For the very flexible, it strengthens the muscles of the legs, arms, shoulders, and back, so the muscles can help hold the joints of the feet, knees, hips, and spine in proper alignment. For the less flexible, the pose provides an excellent stretch for the hamstrings and buttocks. For those with rounded shoulders, it stretches the pectoral muscles on the front of the chest and strengthens the upper back and shoulders.

Notes

- *This pose can be practiced throughout pregnancy to release lower back strain. Late in pregnancy it helps get the weight of the baby off the bladder, to Mom's great relief!*
- *If you have spondylolysis or spondylolisthesis, do not do this pose.*

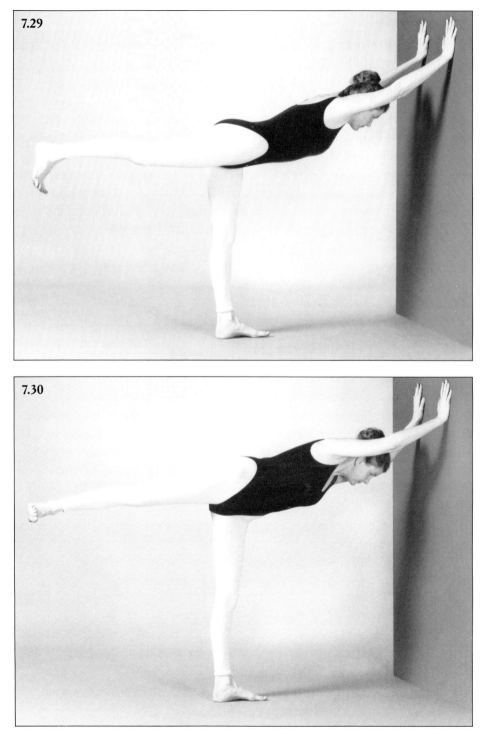

7.29   One-Legged Wall Push
7.30   One-Legged Wall Push, Incorrect

❧

One-Legged Wall Push

Props needed: nonskid surface, wall.

Position and Adjustment. From Wall Push, move your feet closer together so they almost touch. Recheck your foot alignment. On an inhalation, gradually shift the weight onto your left foot. While exhaling, slowly lift your right leg behind you, stretching out through the heel while keeping the knee and leg firm (Figure 7.29). Don't point your toes. Keep pressing into the wall evenly with both hands. Keep your left leg activated by firmly pressing your left heel into the floor.

When your leg is raised, your hips should be in the same position as they were when both feet were on the floor. In other words, don't elevate the right side of the pelvis when you lift the right leg (Figure 7.30, Incorrect). Take care not to overstraighten your elbows. Don't lift your head, but keep it aligned with the spine just as it would be if you were standing up. Imagine that the top of your head is moving toward the wall. Hold the pose for one to three breaths, or as long as you can hold it steadily, without shakiness.

Then, still keeping your right leg actively extended, slowly lower it back to the starting position. Gradually shift the weight back to both feet. Activate your legs and check your foot alignment. Then slowly transfer the weight onto your right foot and stretch out the left leg behind you. Begin with one to three sets for the first few months. Then gradually, over six to eight months, work up to six sets.

Breathing and Imagery. Continue to lengthen your spine with every Total Torso breath. Imagine that the uplifted leg is growing longer from the hip to the heel. Allow the stability of the hands on the wall and the foot on the floor to give a sense of lightness to the lifted leg. Visualize roots extending from the sole of your standing foot into the floor and from the palms of your hands into the wall.

Rationale. This variation of the Wall Push further develops strength in the legs, buttocks, paraspinals, arms, and upper body. It sends a body language message of grace, self-reliance, and capability to the inner self.

Note

• *If you have spondylolysis or spondylolisthesis, do not do this pose.*

❧

Downward-Facing Dog Pose

Props needed: nonskid surface, wall. (As needed:
sturdy chair, two to four blankets.)

Position and Adjustment. This pose resembles the stretch a waking dog performs, with the front legs outstretched, the shoulders lowered, and the pelvis high. If your

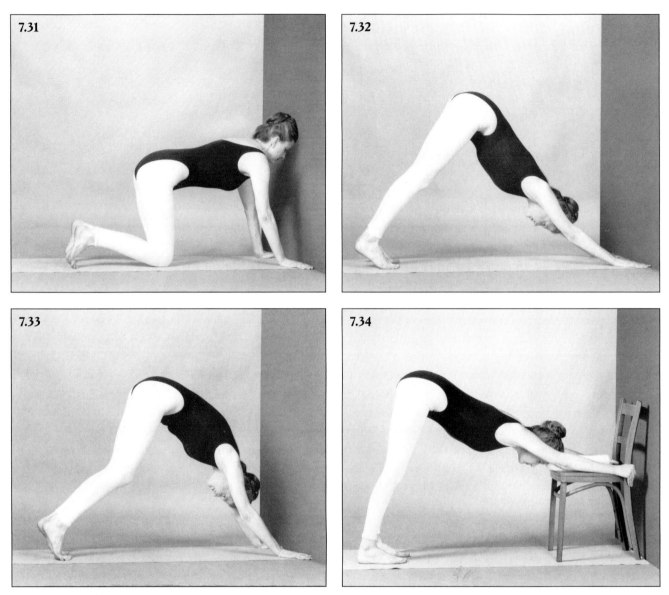

7.31   Downward-Facing Dog Pose, Preparatory Position
7.32   Downward-Facing Dog Pose
7.33   Downward-Facing Dog Pose, Incorrect
7.34   Downward-Facing Dog Pose, Chair Variation

hamstring flexibility evaluation (Figures 4.32, 4.33) has your buttocks more than five inches away from the wall when your legs are up the wall, or if practicing Wall Push requires you to place your hands above shoulder height to maintain good back alignment, postpone Downward-Facing Dog Pose and work on Wall Push for a few months until your hamstring flexibility improves.

Kneel on all fours on a nonskid mat facing a wall (Figure 7.31). Place your hands along the baseboard about shoulder-width apart. Open the space between the index finger and the thumb so that the thumb, like the index finger and middle finger, presses against the baseboard. Position your knees directly under the hips, with the toes tucked under.

On an exhalation, straighten your knees and lift your buttocks toward the ceiling (Figure 7.32). Activate your legs but keep your heels lifted. Push your hands into the wall. If you find that your knees are bent and your back is rounded (Figure 7.33, Incorrect), you are not flexible enough to practice this pose. Try Wall Push instead.

If you are not quite flexible enough for Downward-Facing Dog, yet you want more stretch than Wall Push provides, try this variation: Place a sturdy chair against the wall on your nonskid mat. Place two folded blankets on the chair seat. Perform Downward-Facing Dog Pose with your hands on the back of the chair seat and your forehead resting on the blankets (Figure 7.34).

Elongate your spine from the tip of the tailbone to the crown of the head. Make sure your spine maintains its natural curves, with the lumbar curve neither overarched nor rounded. (You may need another person to help you check your alignment.) Lengthen your legs from the tip of the tailbone to the heels.

Don't let your knees or your elbows overstraighten. Keep your feet parallel, with the weight evenly distributed from the balls of the big toes to the bases of the little toes.

Stay in the pose for one to three breaths, breathing easily. To come out of the pose, bend the knees, returning to all fours. Then rest in Child's Pose (Figure 5.11).

Repeat the pose two or three times for the first one to two months of practice, holding it for one to three breaths each time. During the next six to eight months, increase the time to four to six breaths. Once you can hold the pose for four to six breaths, repeat the pose up to four times.

Breathing and Imagery. Breathe smoothly and gently. Remember not to hold your breath. Imagine roots pulling your hands and feet into the center of the Earth while your tailbone grows toward the sky. Allow your head to be an extension of your spine and your jaw to remain relaxed.

Rationale. Like Wall Push, Downward-Facing Dog Pose is excellent for removing fatigue and releasing tight, tired back muscles. Downward-Facing Dog provides even more stretching and strengthening than Wall Push. For the very flexible, it strengthens the muscles of the legs, arms, shoulders, and back, so the muscles can help hold the joints of the feet, knees, hips, and spine in proper alignment. For the less flexible, it provides an excellent stretch for the hamstrings and buttocks. For those with rounded shoulders, it stretches the pectoral muscles on the front of the chest.

Notes

- *If you have spondylolysis or spondylolisthesis, do not do this pose.*
- *This pose is wonderful throughout pregnancy for back relief and relief of pressure on the bladder. It is especially useful postpartum (as soon as your doctor says you may resume exercise) to counteract the round shoulders that can come from heavy breasts, nursing, and carrying the baby.*

Suggested Routines

Fifteen Minutes

1. One Leg Up, One Leg Out, one minute each side (Figure 6.14)
2. Mountain Pose, activating the legs, one minute (Figures 6.22, 6.23)
3. Standing Twist, two sets, thirty seconds each side (Figures 6.24, 6.25)
4. Wall Push, twenty seconds (Figure 7.25)
5. Triangle Pose, two sets (Figures 7.1–7.5)
6. Revolved Triangle Pose, two sets (Figures 7.7–7.10)
7. Wall Push, twenty seconds (Figure 7.25)
8. Warrior Pose, two sets (Figures 7.16–7.18)
9. Extended Warrior Pose, two sets (Figures 7.22–7.24)
10. Half-Moon Pose, two sets (Figures 7.12–7.14)
11. Downward-Facing Dog Pose (or Wall Push), two times (Figures 7.32, 7.34, 7.25)
12. Child's Pose, two minutes (Figure 5.11)
13. Lying Down with Calves on a Chair, two or more minutes (Figure 5.7)

Twenty Minutes

1. One Leg Up, One Leg Out, one minute each side (Figure 6.14)
2. Mountain Pose, activating the legs, one minute (Figures 6.22, 6.23)
3. Standing Twist, two sets, thirty seconds each side (Figures 6.24, 6.25)
4. Wall Push (or Downward-Facing Dog Pose), thirty seconds (Figures 7.25, 7.32, 7.34)
5. Triangle Pose, three sets, three full breaths on each side (Figures 7.1–7.5)
6. Wall Push (or Downward-Facing Dog Pose), thirty seconds (Figures 7.25, 7.32, 7.34)
7. Revolved Triangle Pose, three sets, three full breaths on each side (Figures 7.7–7.10)
8. Wall Push (or Downward-Facing Dog Pose), thirty seconds (Figures 7.25, 7.32, 7.34)
9. Warrior Pose, three sets, three full breaths on each side (Figures 7.16–7.18)
10. Extended Warrior Pose, three sets, three full breaths on each side (Figures 7.22, 7.23)

11. Wall Push (or Downward-Facing Dog Pose), thirty seconds (Figures 7.25, 7.32, 7.34)

12. Half-Moon Pose, three sets, three full breaths on each side (Figures 7.12–7.14)

13. One-Legged Wall Push, two sets, one to two breaths on each side (Figure 7.29)

14. Supine Child's Pose, two minutes (Figure 5.10)

15. Lying Down with Calves on a Chair, two or more minutes (Figure 5.7)

Notes

- *The order of the standing poses can be varied according to your own needs.*
- *If Triangle Pose is difficult for you, practice Extended Warrior Pose or Revolved Triangle Pose first (or instead). Try Half-Moon Pose before Triangle Pose and see how that feels.*
- *Try this sequence: Half-Moon Pose, One-Legged Wall Push, Warrior Pose, Mountain Pose.*

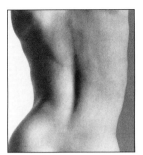

Eight
Sacroiliac Pain and Sciatica

$\mathcal{M}$any people confuse sacroiliac pain with sciatica, because the two conditions share a similar symptom—a pain between the sacrum and the hip on one side. However, the causes of the pain are quite different. Sacroiliac pain is caused by misalignments and prolonged stress on the sacroiliac joints on either side of the base of the spine, where the flat, triangular sacrum joins the other bones of the pelvis. Sciatica is caused by irritation or pressure on the sciatic nerve as it exits the sacrum and passes between layers of the deep buttock muscles and then into the deep muscles of the back of the thigh. With sacroiliac problems, the pain is felt in the SI joint. With sciatica, the pain is felt deep in the buttock in the soft tissues near the SI joint and extends down the leg along the course of the sciatic nerve. It is not unusual for the two conditions to coexist when a tight piriformis muscle pulls the sacrum and the pelvis closer together, simultaneously compressing the sacroiliac joint and the sciatic nerve.

In this chapter, you will learn yoga exercises to help you understand and correct your sacroiliac pain and sciatica.

Sacroiliac Pain

The joints of the bones that form the pelvis, unlike those of the arms, legs, and spine, are held firmly together by ligaments to give great stability and to allow little movement. The sacroiliac (SI) joints are on either side of the base of the spine, where the triangular sacrum meets the wing-shaped ilium bones of the pelvis. To feel your SI joints, hook your thumbs over your hips, thumbs pointing forward and fingertips pointing toward each other below your waist. The tips of your fingers will rest on the slight bulges marking the SI joints (Figure 8.1).

Sacroiliac pain results when slight pelvic rotation, or *torsion*, creates abnormal stresses on the ligaments that join the two bones together. Prolonged stress on the SI ligaments can eventually result in deterioration of the joint surfaces (wear-and-tear arthritis), causing additional pain. Sometimes pain due to SI joint problems is misdiagnosed as lumbar disc disease.

SI pain is usually experienced as a dull ache in the bones above the buttock on one side. But because the nerves in that region are not very specific, pain caused by the SI joint can also be experienced in the groin, back thigh, and lower abdomen. SI pain can be caused by problems in the joint itself or can be caused by nerve signals sent to this area by an injury elsewhere, such as the lower lumbar spine or the hip joint. Usually there is no numbness or tingling, but there may be a dull, heavy feeling in the leg.

Golf, racket sports, and ballet dancing can cause pelvic torsion, placing rotational stress on the SI joint. Asymmetry of the pelvic bones or unequal leg or hamstring length can also cause SI pain: For instance, if the pelvis is tilted to one side, the forces on the two SI joints will be different. Hypermobile SI joints often lead to SI pain in pregnant women, due to the hormone relaxin, which relaxes the ligaments in preparation for childbirth.

Therapeutic exercise for pain in the sacroiliac area is directed at stretching the hamstrings, buttocks, and lower back muscles (which frequently go into spasm when there are SI problems), strengthening all the muscles of the hip girdle to provide support for the pelvis, and strengthening the abdominal muscles to support the front of the spine. To accomplish these goals, you should diligently practice the Home Base and Moving On poses described in Chapters 6 and 7.

Pelvic Torsion as a Cause of Sacroiliac Joint Pain

The source of sacroiliac pain is usually a misalignment of the pelvis. To begin to correct SI pain, you must first be aware that asymmetry exists and that any asymmetrical posture (like sitting with your legs crossed or standing with your weight on one foot) will make the problem worse. If you tend to sleep on your side, it will be helpful to rest your upper knee on a firm pillow.

If the pelvis is rotated to the right or left, there may be tenderness and pain in either sacroiliac joint. You may experience pain in the joint when you hold a heavy object on that side of your body. In order to perform therapeutic exercises for SI pain, you must know which way the pelvis is rotated. If the pelvis is rotated to the right, the right SI joint will protrude more prominently than the left. Similarly, when the pelvis is rotated to the left, the left SI joint will be more prominent. In addition to massaging both SI joints, the following Sacral Rock exercises will help you determine which of your SI joints is more prominent.

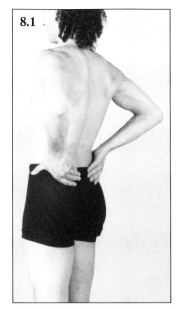

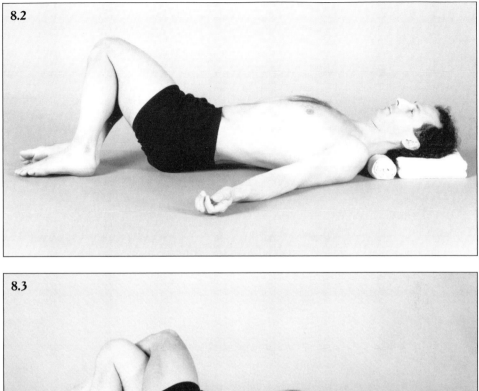

8.1   Locating the SI Joints
8.2   Sacral Rock I
8.3   Sacral Rock II

❀

Sacral Rock I and II

Props needed: head pad, neck support roll.
(As needed: hardcover book or wooden board less
than one-half inch thick.)

Position and Adjustments, Sacral Rock I. Lie on your back on an uncarpeted floor, with your knees bent and your feet parallel on the floor a few inches away from your buttocks. If you do not have an uncarpeted floor, place a hardcover book or thin board (less than one-half inch thick) under your sacrum. Place your neck support roll and head pad behind your neck and head.

Keeping your knees together and your feet on the floor, move your knees slowly to the right six to eight inches (Figure 8.2), and then back to the starting position. Then move your knees slowly to the left and then back. Repeat this at least ten times. Then begin Sacral Rock II.

Sacral Rock II. Cross the left leg over the right, and rock back and forth over the sacrum for thirty seconds (Figure 8.3). Then cross the right leg on top and repeat the exercise.

Breathing and Imagery. Keep your breathing soft, regular, and unforced. Realize that you are giving yourself a massage and relax into it.

Rationale. You are massaging your sacrum and SI joints against the floor. A number of acupressure points are located in this area. Stimulating them sends waves of relaxation up the paraspinal muscles, encouraging them to release their spasm. For this reason, use as firm a surface as you can comfortably tolerate. Notice any asymmetry in the right and left sides of the sacrum during the rocking action. If one SI joint seems to push into the floor more prominently than the other, the pelvis is rotated to that side.

Note

• *Do not practice this pose during the second half of pregnancy.*

❀

Supine Cobbler's Pose

Props needed: head pad, neck support roll.

Position, Adjustment, Breathing, and Imagery. Lie on your back, with appropriate head and neck padding. Place the soles of your feet together, with the knees bent. Have your heels as close to your sitting bones as comfortably possible (Figure 8.4).

While breathing quietly, rock your pelvis slowly in a circle over the sacrum, pressing along its outer edges.

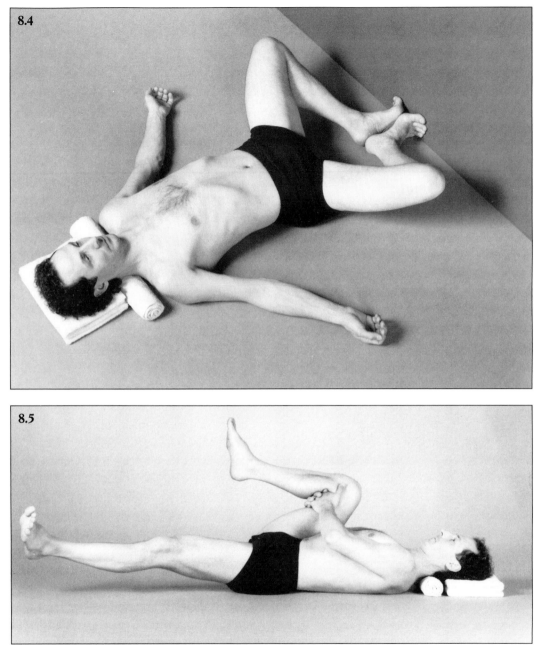

8.4   Supine Cobbler's Pose
8.5   Knee to Chest, Extend Other Leg

Breathe softly and quietly. Imagine a circle around your sacrum and move the weight of your pelvis smoothly around the periphery of that circle. Go around the circle clockwise twice and then counterclockwise twice. Repeat two to four sets.

Rationale. By moving the pelvis in a circle, you can massage the sacrum and determine additional information about the symmetry of the SI joints. With persistence, over many months you can also help the protruding SI joint gradually slip back into alignment. This is also an abdominal muscle strengthener.

Note

• *Do not practice this pose during the second half of pregnancy.*

❧

Knee to Chest, Extend Other Leg

Props needed: head pad, neck support roll.

Position and Adjustment. This pose will help you correct pelvic torsion. Lie on your back with both knees bent, feet on the floor. Use appropriate head and neck padding. Repeat Sacral Rock I and once again note which SI joint is more prominent. If your pelvis is rotated, one SI joint will feel as though it is protruding more into the floor; the other will feel more concave or hollow.

Bend the knee on the side of the more protuberant SI joint toward your chest and hold it there, with your hands holding the back of your thigh (not your knee). Straighten the other leg and lift it three inches from the floor. Stretch out through the heel and then slowly place the leg back on the floor.

Draw the bent leg closer to the chest. Lift the straight leg three inches from the floor, extend it out to the side as far as it will go (Figure 8.5)—for most people, one to two feet—and slowly lower it to the floor. Allow your pelvis to rock to that side as you lower your leg. (The weight of the leg helps to derotate the pelvis.) Then return the leg to the starting position. Once again, draw the bent leg closer to the chest, raise the straight leg three inches from the floor, extend it out to the side, and then set it down.

Then place both feet on the floor with the knees bent and repeat Sacral Rock I to see if the position of the SI joints has changed. If there is a decrease in prominence or tenderness of the protuberant side and a more normal (less caved-in) feeling on the other side, repeat the exercise, again drawing the knee on the side of the more protuberant SI joint toward the chest.

If this adjustment does not make a correction, then try it with a small weight (such as a two-pound bag of beans) held onto your outstretched thigh by an elastic bandage. This will provide more leverage.

If this exercise exaggerates the SI protuberance, try reversing the legs and see if that helps. If you can't correct the pelvic torsion, practice Sacral Rock I and II (Figures 8.2 and 8.3) and Supine Cobbler's Pose (Figure 8.4) for a few months, then try this exercise again.

Check your SI symmetry morning and evening and correct it as necessary with this adjustment. As your leg, back, and buttock muscles gain strength and symmetry through your yoga practice, pelvic torsion will occur less and less often, becoming an exception rather than the rule.

Notes

- *This is an unusual exercise in that it is not repeated on both sides; only the side that gives correction is practiced.*
- *Do not practice this pose during the second half of pregnancy.*

Sciatica

Several nerve roots leave the spinal cord, exit through holes in the sacrum, and combine to form the sciatic nerve, which passes between layers of the deep buttock muscles and then into the deep muscles of the back of the thigh. Pain caused by irritation or pressure on the sciatic nerve anywhere along its course is called sciatica. Characteristically, this pain starts in the buttock and extends down the rear of the thigh and lower leg to the sole of the foot and along the outer side of the lower leg to the top of the foot. Pain may also be felt in the lower back.

A primary cause of sciatica is a herniated or bulging lower lumbar intervertebral disc that compresses one of the nerve roots before it joins the sciatic nerve. Sometimes irritation of a branch of the sciatic nerve in the leg can be so severe as to set up a reflex pain reaction involving the entire length of the nerve—for example, if the nerve is pinched or irritated near the knee, you may feel the pain in the hip and buttock.

Another cause of sciatica is the *piriformis syndrome.* The piriformis muscle extends from the side of the sacrum to the top of the thigh bone at the hip joint, passing over the sciatic nerve en route (Figure 8.6). When a short or tight piriformis is stretched, it can compress and irritate the sciatic nerve. Because the piriformis muscle acts to rotate the leg outward, people who habitually stand with their toes turned out often develop piriformis syndrome, as do runners and cyclists, who overuse and understretch the pirformis muscle.

In order to work therapeutically with sciatica, you must deal with its basic cause. If the source of your sciatica is a bulging disc, the most effective course of treatment is simply to do the Home Base and Moving On exercises in Chapters 6 and 7. If you have a herniated disc or the bulging disc condition is severe, disc surgery might be required.

If the source of your sciatica is a pressure from a short, tight piriformis muscle, the muscle must be gently stretched. The piriformis acts on the leg at the hip joint: It turns the leg out (rotates the leg so that the toes point away from the midline of the body). Spasm of the piriformis muscle can create deep buttock pain that may not be accompanied by sciatica. Both piriformis spasm and piriformis-related sciatica will respond to the following stretch.

❧

Piriformis Stretch

Props needed: blankets.

Position and Adjustment. This stretch is designed to place the piriformis in a stretched position in order to cause it to lengthen over time. Therefore, in someone with sciatic pain due to a short piriformis, this pose will recreate that pain. It is of utmost importance that the pose be adjusted so that you feel a *minimum* amount of discomfort; the muscle should be encouraged to lengthen by gentle stretching. If it is stretched too vigorously, the pain will be unbearable and the muscle will go into spasm, further worsening the condition.

Sit on the corner of a neatly folded blanket four to six inches high, with your knees bent and your feet flat on the floor in front of you. Take your right foot under your left knee and place it on the floor next to your left buttock. Then place your left foot on the floor next to the outside of your right thigh (Figure 8.7). Feel your weight resting equally on both sitting bones. From this base, allow your spine to lengthen upward as you gently lift your breastbone. Stabilize your trunk by holding your left knee with both hands. If your left foot won't reach the floor by your right thigh or if the stretch in your left buttock is too intense, place your left foot next to or in front of your right knee instead.

If the stretch is still too intense or you feel radiating pain down your leg (indicating sciatic nerve irritation) raise the height of the padding beneath your buttocks to decrease the intensity of the stretch to a tolerable level. If you don't feel any stretch in your left buttock, gently pull your left knee across your body toward the right side of your chest.

Stay in the pose for twenty seconds to several minutes. Then repeat on the other side. Do two to four sets. If you can't get comfortable in this pose, practice Crocodile Twist (Figure 6.7) and Revolved Triangle (Figure 7.10) for a few months, then try it again. As your piriformis muscles stretch out over a period of months, gradually decrease the height of your blankets until you can sit on the floor. To make the stretch even more intense, place your hands on the floor in front of you and lean forward from your hips.

Breathing and Imagery. Use the Relaxation Breath. Imagine your spine growing longer. Breathe softness and release into the stretched buttock muscles.

Rationale. This position provides controlled, gentle stretching of the piriformis muscle on the side with the elevated knee. By stretching both sides alternately, you will learn about the differences in tightness and sensitivity on each side.

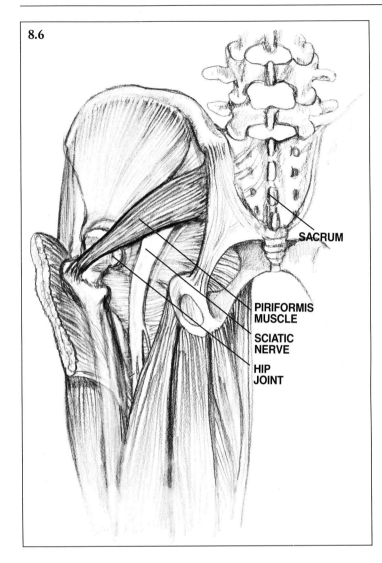

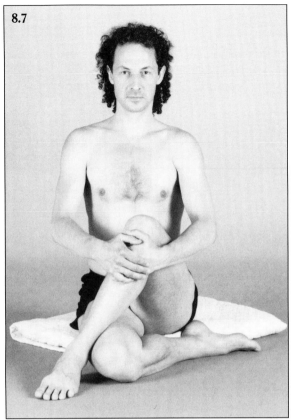

8.6   Sciatic Nerve and Its Relationship to the
       Piriformis Muscle
8.7   Piriformis Stretch

Suggested Routines

If you have pelvic torsion, any of the Relaxation, Home Base, or Moving On routines will be therapeutic for you, but first spend a few minutes using the pelvic torsion correction exercises in this chapter so you start with your pelvis in good alignment. Recheck your pelvic alignment halfway through the routine and, if necessary, do the corrective exercises again before proceeding. At the end of the routine, recheck and realign if necessary.

If you have sciatica due to a tight piriformis or buttock pain due to piriformis spasm, practice Piriformis Stretch (Figure 8.7) at least once a day. This pose can be practiced before Mountain Pose in the Home Base routines and as the second pose in either of the Moving On routines.

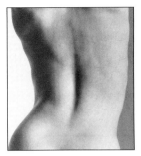

Nine

Rounded Upper Back,
Forward Head Posture, and Neck Pain

*I*f you have forward head posture and a rounded upper back, you are probably well aware that your posture is less than desirable. You may have been told all of your life, as I was, to stand up straight or hold your shoulders up. Unfortunately, following these commands doesn't always help. I am sure the well-meaning relatives and teachers who told me to "hold my shoulders up" had no idea that their advice (which I took literally, raising my still-rounded shoulders toward my ears) would lead to years of neck pain when I reached my forties. By adulthood, tissues and self-image have been molded by years of this posture and improvement does not happen overnight.

If you have had a whiplash injury to you neck, you may have strained or torn muscles and supporting ligaments. Once your doctor has confirmed that you do not have a herniated cervical disc or a vertebral fracture, you can practice these exercises to help relieve muscle spasm and to keep you from further aggravating your neck by poor posture. Remember, your neck will be very sensitive, so practice slowly and gently.

Causes and Effects of Rounded Upper
Back and Forward Head

Posture in which the upper back is abnormally rounded, the chest is collapsed, and the head is forward of the shoulders is frequently associated with depression or a poor self-image. This posture is also seen in older people who have developed crush fractures of the vertebrae due to osteoporosis. Only rarely is it due to congenital bone deformity.

The muscular imbalances associated with forward head and increased rounding of the middle and upper back include weak, overstretched, and overworked muscles in the upper back, overworked neck muscles, and shortened muscles in the upper front chest. This posture can cause physiological disturbances throughout the body. When the upper back is excessively rounded, decreased space is available to the lungs. Therefore, the lungs push the diaphragm downward, decreasing the space in the abdomen. The abdominal contents then push against the abdominal wall, weakening the abdominal muscles, which normally help support the lumbar spine. With the decreased space available in both the chest and abdominal cavities, the circulatory system cannot nourish and cleanse the abdominal organs efficiently, and constipation can result.

The mechanical consequences of this posture reverberate throughout the body. The ability of the upper back to rotate or twist depends on a normal alignment of the vertebrae. (Elderly people sometimes must turn the whole trunk in order to see something behind or to one side of them.) When the thoracic curve is increased, its ability to rotate decreases, and the lower back must provide any necessary rotation. This places excessive demands on the lumbar spine, damaging the lumbar vertebrae and intervertebral discs.

When the head is forward, the normal neck curve becomes flattened. This makes the ligaments taut at first, compressing the vertebrae and limiting motion. As the ligaments become overstretched, instability creates further disc deterioration and reactive bone changes (such as bone spurs).

With the head forward, the upper back muscles must work overtime to support its weight against the pull of gravity, resulting in tension headaches and arthritis of the neck. Sometimes, this posture even causes degeneration and herniation of intervertebral discs in the neck, creating pain, weakness, and numbness in the neck, arm, shoulder, upper back, hand, and fingers. If you develop these symptoms, be sure to consult your physician.

The forward head position strains the lumbar spine, due to weight redistribution and the responses of the lower spinal curves to the change in the cervical curve. It also puts the shoulder joint at a mechanical disadvantage, by moving the collarbone and shoulder blade forward, which can result in bursitis (inflammation of the tissues surrounding the joint) and rotator cuff problems. (The "rotator cuff" is the sleeve of muscle tendons at the shoulder joint which attaches the upper arm bone to the shoulderblades and collarbone. With rounded shoulders and forward head, these tissues are easily injured, torn, inflamed, or swollen.)

Fortunately, you do not have to accept your poor posture (and the physical and psychological pain that go with it). If approached with patience, persistence, gentleness, and attention to alignment, corrective yoga exercises will yield excellent results. Through the exercises in this book, my forward head and stooped shoulder posture have improved so much that I am now more than an inch taller and regularly receive compliments on my posture.

The poses in this chapter focus on the neck and shoulders, but neck pain must be viewed in the context of the entire body and spine, rather than as an isolated problem. To help reduce pain and muscle spasm, begin with the exercises in this chapter and then work on the Home Base and Moving On poses (Chapters 6 and 7) to get at the roots of your posture problem.

Neck Stretches

Warning: Traditional head-rolling exercises can be hazardous. Yes, I know you've seen people rolling their heads around on their necks in exercise classes and books for years. You've even tried doing it and it felt good. But because head-rolling exercises do not honor the functional limitations of the cervical (neck) spine, they can be counterproductive.

Unlike the hip joint, which has a ball-and-socket configuration, the facet joints of the neck vertebrae have flat surfaces that glide on each other only when movement is in the plane of the surfaces. If the neck joints were of the ball-and-socket type, head rolling exercises would be appropriate. But because they are not, the outer edges of the facet joints grate against each other when they are forced to approximate this type of rotational movement. This harmful action can cause arthritic changes and muscle spasm.

The following well-aligned neck exercises will stretch and relax neck muscles within the limitations dictated by the anatomy of the cervical vertebrae. These neck stretches work on the small muscles of the neck and on the shoulder girdle muscles where they attach to the cervical spine. These muscles are called upon to work overtime in forward head posture and greatly appreciate being stretched to allow better circulation and improved posture. (These exercises can also be performed standing, but they are easier to learn while sitting.)

The neck stretches should create no pain. If you have a history of neck injury, spurs on the cervical vertebrae, a herniated cervical intervertebral disc, arthritis of the cervical spine, or pain or numbness radiating into the neck or down the arm, proceed with great caution with these stretches. They can be beneficial for all of these conditions if used properly, but you must take special care to avoid creating pain or numbness. Always move gently and slowly, floating the head and neck into position. If discomfort occurs only in the final position, do not go all the way into the pose.

❧

Sitting Well

Props needed: sturdy chair with a firm, flat seat.
(As needed: books, blankets, beanbag.)

Position and Adjustment. Choose a sturdy chair with a firm, flat seat. The height of the chair should be such that when you are sitting on the forward third of the seat, your thighs can be parallel to the floor and your knees exactly over your ankles (Figure 9.1). If the seat is so high that your feet cannot touch the floor, place books under your feet. If the seat is so low that your knees are higher than your hip joints (Figure 9.2, Incorrect), sit on a folded blanket (Figure 9.3). Otherwise, your sitting position will create stress in your lower back and make good posture difficult.

Take a few moments to locate the top of your head, the point at which a line drawn across the top of your head from one ear hole to the other intersects a line drawn up the center of your face to the top of your head. (You can use a couple of strings to find the exact spot.) Press on this spot so that you can feel it during the rest of this exercise. Practicing this pose with a bean bag on the top of your head will teach you to lengthen your spine straight up.

Sit on your sitting bones, not your tailbone and sacrum. Make sure that your weight remains equal on the right and the left sitting bones. To avoid slumping, allow your breastbone to gently lift, but without overarching your lower back. Sit in this position, concentrating on your breathing, imagery, and alignment, for one to three minutes at least once a day and as often as possible during daily activities.

Breathing and Imagery. Imagine that your sitting bones are sending roots down toward the center of the Earth, holding your torso steadily in place. Imagine that the top of your head is a lofty treetop reaching for the sun. With each inhalation and exhalation, feel lightness in your spine as it elongates upward from its steady base. Keep your chin level, neither elevated nor lowered. Release the muscles at the base of your skull. Keep your neck and shoulders soft and relaxed, with your shoulders dropping away from your ears.

Another useful image is to visualize a cloud beneath your skull where it joins the spinal column. With each inhalation, let the cloud gradually and softly expand. With each exhalation, let your head float upward off of the spine.

Rationale. Sitting erect strengthens the upper back muscles that support the neck. This posture puts the head, neck, and shoulders in the proper alignment for the stretches that follow.

Ear to Shoulder I

Props needed: sturdy chair with a firm, flat seat.
(As needed: books, folded blanket.)

Position and Adjustment. Sit in a sturdy chair with a firm seat, as in the preceding pose. Sit forward on the chair seat, with your weight equally distributed on the two sitting bones. Feel a strong connection of the sitting bones with the chair seat. Feel your spine stretch from the sitting bones toward a point beyond the top of your head. Remember

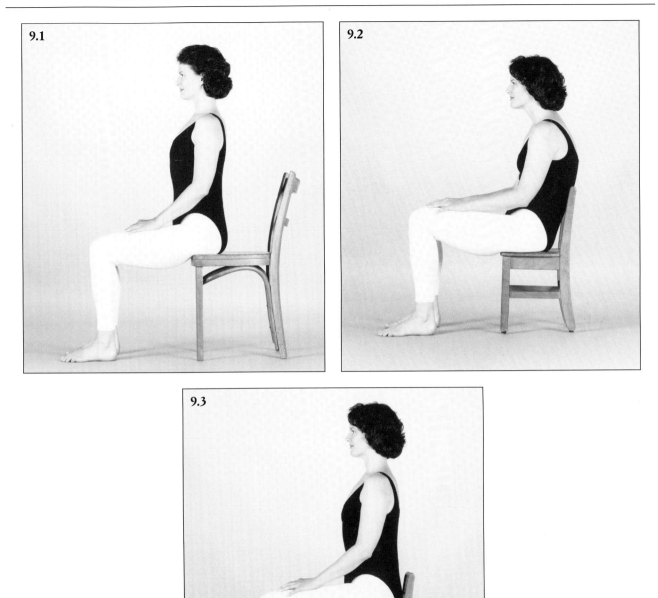

9.1   Sitting Well
9.2   Sitting, Incorrect Chair Height
9.3   Sitting, Corrected

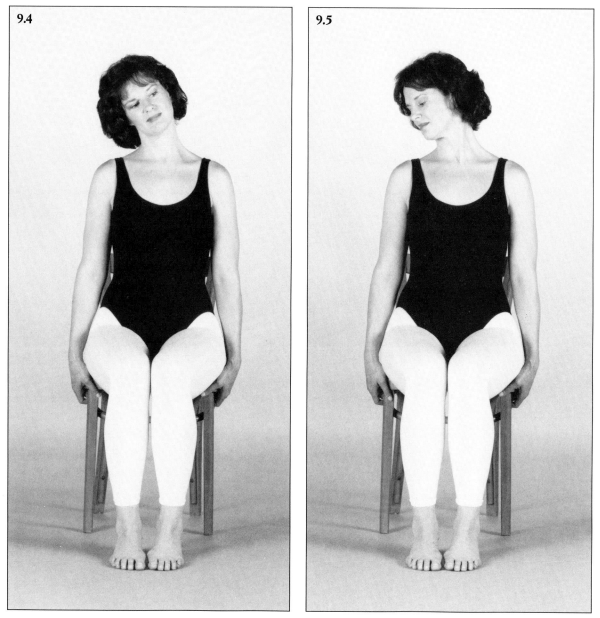

9.4   Ear to Shoulder I
9.5   Ear to Shoulder II

to keep your breastbone lifting without overarching your lower back. For several breaths, allow your spine to feel longer than you think it is.

Imagine a soft, fluffy cloud between the top of your spinal column and the base of your skull. Let this cloud float your head up off of the spine. This is more of a non-action than an action, an allowing rather than a doing. The chin should stay level (neither elevated nor lowered) as the entire head floats up. Release any tension in your shoulders.

Inhale, and on the exhalation, allow your head to float up, sideways, and down, so that your right ear moves closer to your right shoulder (Figure 9.4). Don't raise your shoulder to your ear or elevate your chin. Keep your eyes open and looking down. Keep your jaw relaxed. Stay in this position for twenty to forty seconds (about three to five breaths).

Then float your head back up to the starting position. Again, feel your connection with your sitting bones and let your spine lengthen upward.

Then float your head up, sideways, and down to the left side, bringing your left ear closer to the left shoulder without elevating the chin or the left shoulder. Do two to four sets.

Breathing and Imagery. As your ear travels up, sideways, and down toward your shoulder, imagine that your ear is a feather, blown up and sideways by a gentle breeze, then floating softly to the ground. Breathe softly and quietly, so that the quality of your breath gives gentleness to the stretch.

Ear to Shoulder II

Prop needed: sturdy chair.
(As needed: books, blanket.)

Position and Adjustment. The first part of this stretch is the same as in the preceding pose. Once you have held the ear-to-shoulder position for at least twenty seconds, then gradually, in steps, turn your head so that your eyes are looking toward your armpit (Figure 9.5). Stop two times along the way to inhale into the area where you feel the most stretch and exhale as you allow the stretched area to release. Each time you pause, hold that position for at least twenty seconds before going further into the stretch. Make sure that both shoulders stay low, away from your ears. Remember to keep your jaw relaxed and your eyes open and looking down. Float your head back up to the starting position. Then repeat on the other side. Do three to six sets, remembering to float your head back up to the starting position after each stretch.

Breathing and Imagery. Use the Relaxation Breath. See the muscles along the side of your neck becoming longer, softer, and more free. See the distance between your ear and your shoulder gradually increase.

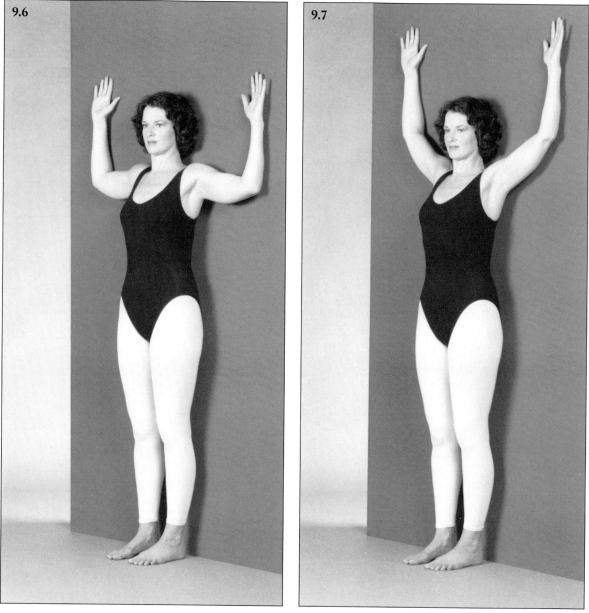

9.6   Arm Raises, Starting Position
9.7   Arm Raises, Final Position

Rationale. The Ear to Shoulder stretches lengthen the muscles that connect the head to the neck and shoulders. As they lengthen, the space between your vertebrae will increase and you will find it easier to realign your head and shoulders. With more space between the vertebrae, there will be less stress on the cervical discs and facet joints.

Poses for the Upper Back and Shoulders

Arm Raises

Props needed: wall. (As needed: two cans of peas.)

Position and Adjustment. Stand erect with your back to the wall, your heels six to eight inches from the baseboard and your feet hip-width apart. Lean against the wall with your shoulders and buttocks. Make sure that your breastbone is lifted but your lower back is not overarched.

Raise your bent arms so that each upper arm extends along the wall in line with the shoulder and each elbow is bent ninety degrees (Figure 9.6). Keeping your elbows and wrists in contact with the wall as long as possible, slowly reach for the ceiling until both elbows are straight, as if you were flying. (Figure 9.7). Keep your shoulders lowered away from your ears. Don't allow your back to overarch.

Slowly lower your arms back to the bent-elbow position. Repeat five times. If this is easy and painless, hold a one-pound weight in each hand (soft drinks or cans of peas work quite well as weights). Gradually increase the number of repetitions until you are able to do twenty-five.

Breathing and Imagery. Breathe gently and easily. Don't hold your breath. Feel the muscles below your shoulder blades working and becoming stronger to help you overcome round shoulders. When your arms are extended over your head, feel as though you could fly.

Rationale. The muscles of the upper back and shoulders help hold the upper body erect. When the shoulders are rounded and the head is forward, they must overwork in an abnormally elongated position that puts them at a biomechanical disadvantage. They benefit from strengthening in a position of good posture.

Notes

• *If either of these positions causes pain in the shoulder joints, decrease the length of time you hold the position or the number of repetitions. If that does not help, delete the straight-arm portion and work only on the bent-elbow pose for a few months while working on general posture improvement. It may take some time*

151

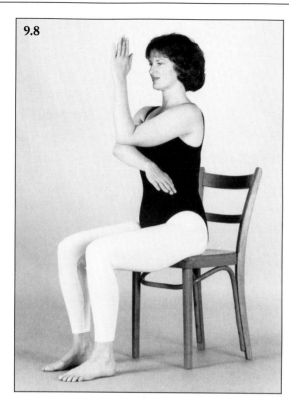

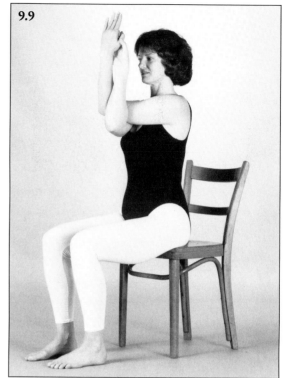

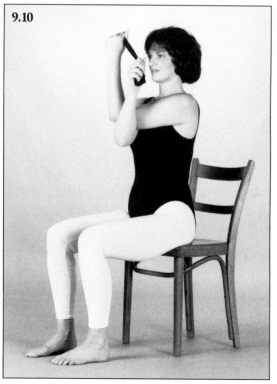

9.8   Entwine the Forearms, Going into the Pose
9.9   Entwine the Forearms, Final Position
9.10 Entwine the Forearms, Variation for Limited Flexibility

*for people with shoulder injuries to be able to lift the arms over the head
without pain.*

- *If your wrists or elbows do not touch the wall, keep them as close to the wall
as you comfortably can. They will move closer over time and with perseverance.*

❖

Entwine the Forearms

Props needed: sturdy chair. (As needed: books,
blanket, beanbag; belt, sock, or small towel.)

Position and Adjustment. Sit in a chair, using good sitting posture, as
described in preceding poses. (Putting a beanbag on top of your head will help you improve
your posture.) Be aware of the weight of your body on your sitting bones, and lengthen your
torso up from the top of your head, while keeping your jaw relaxed, your shoulders low,
your chin level, and your eyes open and looking down.

Place your left arm, with the elbow bent at a right angle, in front of the center
of your chest, with your elbow at the height of your middle chest (Figure 9.8). Stretch your
right arm out straight, take it under your upper left arm, and then reach back toward your
left forearm to entwine the arms so that the fingers of your right hand touch your left palm
(Figure 9.9). If your hands don't meet, hold a belt, sock, or small towel in your left hand
and grasp it with your right hand at a comfortable height (Figure 9.10). Feel the stretch
across your upper back. Keep your weight evenly distributed on your sitting bones. To
increase the stretch, raise your elbows an inch or two, and hold this position while continuing to breathe quietly. Hold at least twenty seconds at each position.

Repeat on the other side. Note the differences from one side to the other.

Breathing and Imagery. Use the Relaxation Breath, pausing at the end of each
exhalation. With each inhalation, imagine that your upper back is broadening. With each
exhalation, see the upper back muscles becoming soft and pliable.

Rationale. This stretch is helpful when the upper back muscles (especially the
rhomboids, which attach the shoulder blades to the spine) go into spasm. Because it exaggerates the roundedness of the shoulders, it should be used only occasionally, when the
upper back muscles are painful.

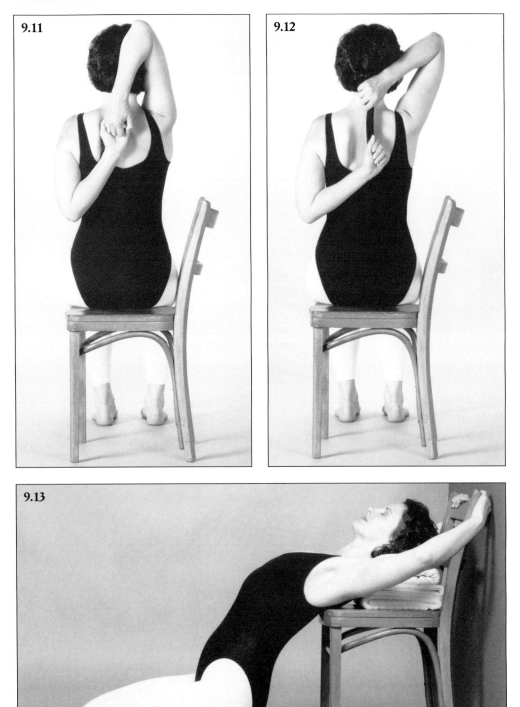

9.11 One Elbow Up, One Elbow Down, Final Position

9.12 One Elbow Up, One Elbow Down, Variation for Limited Flexibility

9.13 Kneeling Backbend, Passive

❦

One Elbow Up, One Elbow Down

Prop needed: chair. (As needed: blanket, books, long
sock or hand towel.)

Position and Adjustment. Begin in a chair in your best sitting posture, equalizing your weight on both sitting bones and lengthening up from the top of your head. Keep your shoulders low, chin level, jaw relaxed, and eyes open and looking down toward the lower eyelids. Stretch your right arm straight up over your head and then bend your elbow so that your palm touches your back between the shoulder blades.

Stretch your left arm straight back behind your body and then bend the elbow, placing your hand in the middle of your back above your waist, palm out. If possible, clasp the two hands together (Figure 9.11). If the fingers just barely touch or if it is impossible to bring your hands together, hold the sock or towel in your right hand and grasp it with your left (Figure 9.12). Do not allow the good alignment of your head to change or your lower back to overarch.

Now stretch up through the right elbow and down through the left elbow. Hold for at least twenty seconds. Repeat on the other side. Observe any differences in the two sides. Do two to four sets.

Caution. Remember to keep your jaw relaxed. Resist the impulse to overarch your lower back or shift your weight to one side.

Breathing and Imagery. Breathe gently and softly. With each inhalation, lengthen your upper elbow toward the ceiling and your lower elbow toward the floor. Visualize your spine lengthening from your sitting bones up through the top of your head.

Rationale. This stretch works on the muscles that control the shoulder joint. It lengthens the muscles and develops greater freedom of movement, so the rounded shoulders and forward head can gradually return to a more normal alignment.

❦

Kneeling Backbend

Props needed: wall, sturdy chair, four blankets.
(As needed: socks, belt.)

Position and Adjustment. Place the chair with its back against the wall. Place a neatly folded blanket on the chair seat so it hangs over the front edge enough to pad it. Place the other folded blankets in a stack on the rear of the seat.

Kneel on a blanket with your back to the chair, knees hip-width apart. If your knees are uncomfortable, pad them by making an extra fold in your blanket.

Passive Variation. Lean back so that the edge of the chair seat presses just below your shoulder blades. Let your head rest on the blankets (Figure 9.13). If it won't reach, fold the blankets to make them higher. Hold the back of the chair, elbows pointing to either side. If there is pain in either knee, come out of the pose, insert a sock in the bend of the knee, and try again. If your knees tend to separate, fasten a belt around your upper thighs. Rest in the pose with your hips sitting on your heels for twenty seconds to several minutes. Then rest in Child's Pose (Figure 9.16).

Active Variation 1. Lift your hips while pressing your knees, shins, and feet into the floor (Figure 9.14). Hold for several breaths, then rest in Child's Pose (Figure 9.16).

Active Variation 2. From the starting position sitting on your heels, reach behind you and firmly grasp the front of the chair seat. Press strongly down with your hands, feet, and shins to lift your hips and straighten your arms. Keep pressing down with your hands and shins to open up your chest, roll your shoulders back, and move your hips forward (Figure 9.15). Keep looking forward—don't throw your head back. If your lower back complains, come out of the pose by sitting back down on your heels. Try it again, this time being careful to keep the pubic bone moving toward the navel as you lift your hips. If your upper back muscles cramp, sit on your heels and hug yourself until it stops. If your feet cramp, tuck your toes under.

Hold the pose for several breaths. Then rest in Child's Pose (Figure 9.16).

Breathing and Imagery. For the passive variation, use the Relaxation Breath. For the active variations, breathe naturally with your eyes open and looking downward. Don't hold your breath. Visualize your chest opening up to receive more oxygen. See your rounded shoulders releasing their stiffness. See your heart becoming more open and receptive.

Rationale. This pose helps lengthen the pectoral (front chest) muscles and the muscles between the ribs so that head and upper body carriage can improve. The second active variation also strengthens the upper back muscles.

Notes

- *During the first half of pregnancy, practice only the passive variation of this pose.*
- *Do not practice this pose at all during the second half of pregnancy.*

❀

Supported Supine Resting Pose

Props needed: three blankets, many towels
or washcloths.

Position and Adjustment. If your upper back is severely rounded, comfortably propping yourself in a supine position requires a firm blanket and a good supply of towels and patience. If the curve is longstanding, the upper back will not flatten out on the floor; therefore props must be used to comfortably support your spine and shoulders as they are now. As your posture improves in the coming months, the thickness of the props may be reduced.

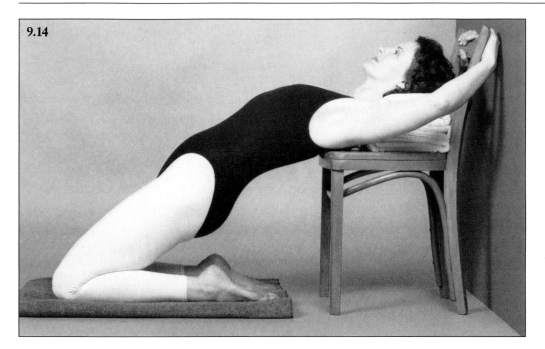

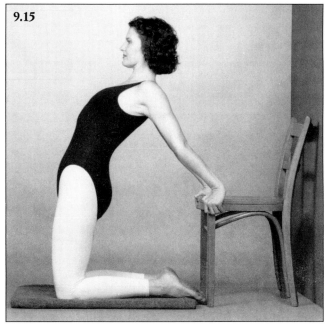

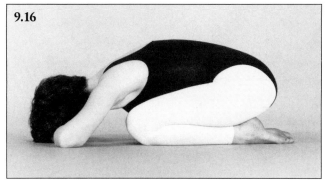

9.14   Kneeling Backbend, Variation 1
9.15   Kneeling Backbend, Variation 2
9.16   Child's Pose

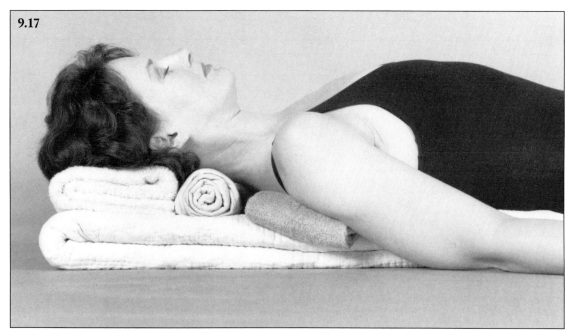

9.17 **Supported Supine Resting Pose**

Neatly fold a firm blanket to a thickness of one to two inches and a width of twelve inches. To support your shoulder blades, place one or more folded washcloths or towels on either side of the midline of the blanket. Sit on the floor near one end of the blanket. Using your hands for support, lay your torso down on the blanket, with your shoulder blades resting on the towels. Support your neck with a firmly rolled towel and your head with a folded towel (Figure 9.17). (Refer to the detailed description of neck support roll and head pad in Chapter 5, "Relaxation Techniques." Also see Figures 5.3–5.5.)

You may need to use several additional folded towels to elevate and support your head and shoulders. If the pressure of your spine on the blanket is uncomfortable, use two folded blankets, side by side, to create a groove within which your spine can be suspended.

Adjust the thickness of each prop until you are *absolutely* comfortable. Readjust props during the pose if more support is required under your neck, head, shoulders, and shoulder blades as muscles relax.

Hold the position only as long as it is comfortable. Start with one to two minutes, gradually building up to five to ten minutes or more.

Breathing and Imagery. Use the Relaxation Breath. See your lungs expanding to receive the breath. See healing air flowing to each cell, bringing it energy and strength and helping it to heal.

Rationale. In this supported restorative pose, a passive stretch for the pectoral muscles helps promote better posture. The firm support of the props allows muscles to release and lengthen. Relaxation can begin to heal the body and spirit. The chest is no longer collapsed, breathing is easier, and circulation to the abdominal organs is improved.

Note

• *Do not practice this pose during the second half of pregnancy.*

Sleeping Positions and Neck Pain

The lessons you have learned about maintaining and supporting your normal spinal curves can help heal your neck even while you sleep. If your neck is painful upon waking, it is a good bet that it will respond nicely to better alignment and support while you sleep. Here are a few tips:

• A firm mattress helps all types of sleepers.
• Sleeping on your stomach can be a real problem if you have neck pain, especially if you have a soft mattress. If you must sleep this way, put your chest, neck, and head on top of a large pillow. You may feel better if your entire torso, neck, and head are on top of two pillows.
• For sleeping on the back, use the same neck support roll and head pad that

you made for your yoga practice (see Figures 5.3–5.5). Just slip them inside a pillowcase for sleeping (or make another set to keep on the bed). If you have a cervical pillow that has totally relieved your early morning neck discomfort, stick with it. Most cervical pillows, however, are too soft to provide adequate support. Also, they are made for the average neck, so they will not fit you as well as the roll and pad you create specifically for yourself.

- If you sleep lying on your side, you must fill in the space between the bed and your shoulder, the side of your head, and your neck, in order to support your head and neck. Otherwise you will sleep with a kink in your cervical spine. The supporting neck roll and head pad for lying on your side must be thicker than one for lying on your back (Figure 11.13).

Have several folded towels available to fill in the space between the bed and the side of your head and neck. Try different thicknesses until you find the most comfortable height. Make sure that your neck is supported also; don't leave it hanging in space between your head and shoulder.

Learn to sleep directly on the end of your shoulder, not with the shoulder rounded forward so that you lie on your shoulder blade. Before you put your weight on your shoulder, move it down away from your ear (to make your neck feel longer).

Once you have arranged all this, turn your attention to your top arm. If you do not support the top arm, it will pull on your neck all night, giving you a painful message the next morning. Use a fat pillow to support this arm while you sleep.

- If you sleep in more than one position, have proper pillows and padding for your favorite positions handy. The relief they provide will remind you to reach for them as you change positions. A number of my neck patients who are restless sleepers have found considerable relief by sleeping in a cervical foam collar. This provides neck support as you continue to change positions during the night. (Soft cervical collars are available at surgical supply stores for about fifteen dollars.)

Suggested Routines

Fifteen Minutes (for neck and upper back)
1. Sitting Well, one minute (Figure 9.1)
2. Ear to Shoulder I, three sets (Figure 9.4)
3. Ear to Shoulder II, three sets (Figure 9.5)
4. Arm Raises, four times (Figures 9.6, 9.7)
5. Entwine the Forearms, two sets (Figures 9.8–9.10)
6. One Elbow Up, One Elbow Down, two sets (Figures 9.11, 9.12)
7. Kneeling Backbend, Active Variation 1 or 2, one minute (Figures 9.14–9.16)

8. Kneeling Backbend, Passive Variation, one minute (Figures 9.13, 9.16)

9. Supported Supine Resting Pose, one or more minutes (Figure 9.17)

10. Elbows on the Table, one or more minutes (Figure 5.8)

Twenty Minutes (for neck and upper back, combined with Home Base poses)

1. Supine Pelvic Tilt, with attention to pressing the head, shoulders, and arms to the floor, three times (Figure 6.1)

2. One Leg Up, One Leg Out, one set, one minute each side (Figures 6.14, 6.15)

3. Sitting Well, Ear to Shoulder I and II, three minutes (Figures 9.1, 9.4, 9.5)

4. Mountain Pose, activating the legs, one minute (Figures 6.22, 6.23)

5. Supine Knee-Chest Twist, Variation 1, two sets (Figure 6.5)

6. Supine Knee-Chest Twist, Variation 2, two sets (Figure 6.6)

7. Crocodile Twist, two sets (Figure 6.7)

8. Standing Twist, two sets (Figures 6.24, 6.25)

9. Passive Back Arch, one minute (Figures 6.8–6.11)

10. Easy Bridge Pose, three times (Figures 6.12, 6.13)

11. Kneeling Backbend, Active Variation 1 or 2, one minute (Figures 9.14–9.16)

12. Kneeling Backbend, Passive Variation, one minute (Figures 9.13, 9.16)

13. All Fours, Variation 1, two sets (Figures 6.19, 6.20)

14. All Fours, Variation 2, two sets (Figures 6.19, 6.21)

15. Supported Supine Resting Pose, two or more minutes (Figure 9.17)

Twenty Minutes (for neck and upper back, combined with Home Base and Moving On poses)

1. Supine Pelvic Tilt, with attention to pressing the shoulders, head, and arms to the floor, three times (Figure 6.1)

2. Mountain Pose, one minute (Figures 6.22, 6.23)

3. Standing Twist, two sets (Figures 6.24, 6.25)

4. Wall Push or Downward-Facing Dog Pose, thirty seconds (Figures 7.25, 7.32, 7.34)

5. Triangle Pose, three sets (Figures 7.1–7.5)

6. Wall Push or Downward-Facing Dog Pose, thirty seconds (Figures 7.25, 7.32, 7.34)

7. Revolved Triangle Pose, three sets (Figures 7.7–7.10)

8. Wall Push or Downward-Facing Dog Pose, thirty seconds (Figures 7.25, 7.32, 7.34)

9. Warrior Pose, three sets (Figures 7.16–7.18)

10. Wall Push or Downward-Facing Dog Pose, thirty seconds (Figures 7.25, 7.32, 7.34)

11. Half-Moon Pose, three sets (Figures 7.12–7.14)

12. One-Legged Wall Push, two sets (Figure 7.29)

13. Kneeling Backbend, Active Variation 1 or 2, one minute (Figures 9.14–9.16)

14. Kneeling Backbend, Passive Variation, one minute (Figures 9.13, 9.16)
15. Supine Child's Pose, one minute (Figure 5.10)
16. Supported Supine Resting Pose, one or more minutes (Figure 9.17)
17. Child's Pose (Figure 5.11) or Elbows on the Table (Figure 5.8), one or more minutes

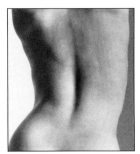

Ten

Scoliosis

$\mathcal{S}$ometimes back pain is associated with abnormal side-to-side curves of the spine, referred to as *scoliosis*. In what is called *true scoliosis*, these curves are caused by abnormal development of the muscles and bones of the spine, and cannot be easily corrected (although yoga postures can relieve pain, prevent the condition from worsening, and sometimes partially reverse it). In *functional scoliosis*, the curves are caused by variables outside of the spine itself, such as asymmetrical work or a short leg that tilts the pelvis to one side: If the imbalances associated with this condition are corrected, the scoliosis will disappear.

Functional Scoliosis

Functional scoliosis can be caused by a variety of factors, including back spasms and real or apparent leg-length differences.

Real leg-length difference. If one leg is longer than the other, the pelvis will tilt to one side. To keep the head level, the body adjusts by curving the spine to balance the pelvic tilt. Diagnosis of this condition requires careful measurements or leg X-rays.

Muscles on the concave side of the curved spine are shortened; on the convex side they are elongated. Those with a true leg-length discrepancy must practice exercises to balance the muscles on either side of the spine, such as the standing poses described in Chapter 7. During daily activities a lift in the shoe of the short leg will also help decrease the imbalance. However, unless the leg-length difference is two or more inches, the exercises in this book should still be practiced barefoot. When needed (as in Mountain Pose, Figure 6.22, for example), a board can be placed under the foot of the short leg to level the pelvis.

Apparent leg-length difference (functional short leg). Even if the leg bones are of equal length, lateral spinal curvature can result if the joints of legs and feet are not used symmetrically. If one foot flattens, one ankle collapses inward, one knee is straightened too far or incompletely straightened, or one hip joint is slightly flexed, the length of that leg will seem different from the other. The same sorts of imbalances in the muscle and bones of the spine can occur with functional as with real leg-length difference.

Working with functional leg-length discrepancy requires recognizing the misalignment of the feet or legs. Chapters 6 and 7 provide Home Base and Moving On exercises to strengthen the muscles that support the arch to correct flat foot, to stretch the back leg muscles for full straightening of the knee, to balance the muscles that control the knee joint to prevent hyperextension, and to stretch the hip flexors for full extension of the hip.

The key to working with functional leg-length discrepancy is to realize that you do not have to allow the abnormality to continue. At first, correction of the misalignment requires constant attention and awareness. Later, as new habits of movement develop and muscles reset their resting lengths, proper alignment can be maintained more easily.

Back spasm scoliosis. So-called back spasm scoliosis occurs when the muscles on one side of the spine go into spasm (prolonged painful contraction) as a result of acute back injury or disc herniation. The muscle contraction on one side of the spine causes the appearance of a curvature, which reverts to normal when the muscles are relaxed. The poses in Chapter 5, "Relaxation Techniques," will help treat back spasms. The Home Base and Moving On poses will help prevent the injuries that lead to back spasm scoliosis.

True Scoliosis

The most common form of true scoliosis is *idiopathic adolescent scoliosis*, which occurs during the growth spurt for unknown reasons. True scoliosis can also result when polio paralyzes the muscles acting on one side of the spine. Or it can be caused by *hemivertebrae,* a condition in which only half of the vertebra develops, resulting in a wedge-shaped vertebra that is of normal or nearly normal thickness on one side and much less-than-normal thickness on the other side.

Regardless of the cause of the scoliosis, the abnormal spinal curves are associated with imbalances in the paraspinal muscles, which run parallel to the spine and act upon it. The muscles on the long aspect (convexity) of the curvature become overstretched and weakened. The muscles on the short aspect (concavity) of the curvature become overworked and tightened (Figure 10.1). This muscle imbalance causes further distortion of the spinal column and an uneven weight distribution over all of the facet joints. The facet joints on the inner aspect of the curve are damaged by chronically working under increased pressure.

10.1

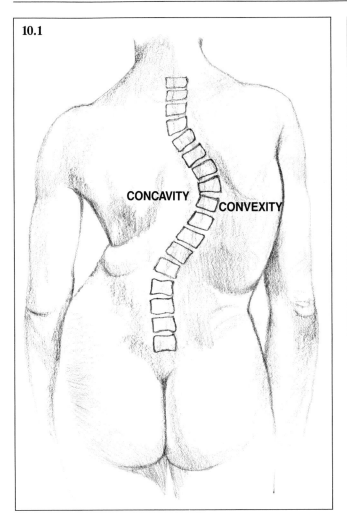

CONCAVITY   CONVEXITY

10.2

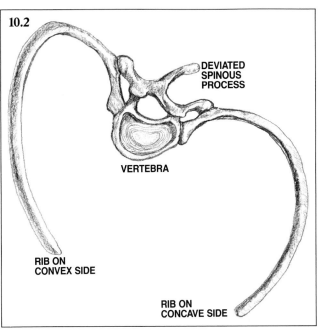

DEVIATED
SPINOUS
PROCESS

VERTEBRA

RIB ON
CONVEX SIDE

RIB ON
CONCAVE SIDE

10.1   Scoliosis, Spinal Concavity and Convexity. Adapted with
permission from CIBA-Geigy, from drawings by Frank
Netter, M.D.

10.2   Rib Asymmetry. Adapted with permission from CIBA-
Geigy, from drawings by Frank Netter, M.D.

In both structural and functional scoliosis, the uneven demands on the facet joints can cause wear-and-tear arthritis and can lead to degeneration of the intervertebral discs.

Practicing Yoga with a Helper

If you have scoliosis, it is best to practice yoga with a helper, although you can also benefit from working alone. Your helper could be a yoga teacher, friend, or family member. If you have a friend with scoliosis, work together. You'll both understand your backs much better if you alternate "doing" and "helping."

People with scoliosis usually have a distorted sense of what constitutes a straight spine. (The body's inner balancing mechanism tells us that we are "straight" when our eyes are level with the horizon. A person with scoliosis will unconsciously distort the whole body in an attempt to level the eyes.) Your helper can tell you when you are actually straightening your spine by providing visual and tactile advice about how your spine should be moving. If you are not experienced in therapeutic yoga and wish to help someone with scoliosis, you should carefully read this chapter and Chapter 4, "Assessing Your Flexibility and Alignment," especially the section on scoliosis.

Although scoliosis is defined as an abnormal lateral (side-to-side) curvature in the spine, there are many variations on this theme. Some people have a single lateral curve. Others have a double curve. Some even have a triple curve. The side-to-side curve is complicated by rotation of part of the spine. It is important for the helper to look carefully at the spine and assess the curves. (It is not necessary to have X-rays to assess the curves, but it does help to wear a bathing suit or a low-backed leotard so your back is visible.) It may be helpful for the helper to use a marking pen to place a dotted line following the spinous processes of the vertebrae. The helper can locate the spinous processes either by sight or by touch, with the practitioner bending forward while seated in a sturdy chair. (The entire spine should be as rounded as possible during this demonstration, to make the spinous processes more prominent.)

Advice to Helpers

If you are helping someone with scoliosis, you will probably notice that your friend's upper back appears rounded. Carefully examine the upper back to see whether this rounded appearance is due to a rounded upper spine or to a rib prominence on one side. In idiopathic adolescent scoliosis (the type of scoliosis that begins in adolescence and usually affects females), the thoracic spine is usually *not* abnormally rounded, but flattened and rotated. (In some cases, the thoracic curve will actually be concave, like the lumbar spine, rather than convex.) The upper back appears rounded because the ribs protrude on one side. When the thoracic vertebrae rotate, the spinous processes move toward one side, and the ribs attached to the vertebrae will protrude in back on the other side (Figure 10.2). Not only is the thoracic curve flattened, but so is the lumbar curve. Once you get a better understanding of what is happening in the spine, you will better understand how to guide your friend toward a more normal alignment.

Many people with scoliosis have problems related to the prolonged effects of gravity on a spine that does not distribute weight optimally. Much of the musculoskeletal pain is related to collapse and loss of space around joints and moving parts. For this reason the hanging poses in this chapter give great pain relief. My students with scoliosis all say hanging poses are their favorites.

Another area prone to pain is the shoulder blade that has been displaced upward by the rib prominence. Help the practitioner keep this shoulder blade from riding up and destroying the normal functioning of that shoulder joint.

Yet another vulnerable area is the inner side, or concavity, of the side-to-side spinal curvature. Compression of joints, muscles, and nerves occurs here. Learning to increase space in the concavity can help the student.

Just as the concave (inner) side of the lateral spinal curve can create pain due to collapse, the convex (outer) aspect of this curve can be painful because of overstretching. You can help the practitioner adjust each movement to avoid either overstretching or compression in the area. This is usually a challenging endeavor, but a worthwhile one, as it teaches the person with scoliosis that it is possible to change movement habits and avoid pain.

❧

Hanging

Props needed: exercise horse, table, or counter; sturdy
chair, nonskid surface, partner. (As needed: blankets.)

Position and Adjustment. This pose can be done over a table or counter of the appropriate height. The weight of your torso is suspended from your thighs, with your hips bent at ninety degrees. Your folded arms should not touch the floor. If the table is not high enough, place folded blankets on it.

To get into the pose, place the chair about a foot from the table, with the seat facing the table. Sit on the table, then use the strength of your arms to let yourself down onto your side on the tabletop. Roll over onto your belly and slowly scoot yourself to the edge of the table. While your helper holds your thighs or calves, hold onto the chair seat and gradually move your trunk off the table. Release your hold on the chair and put your hands on the floor. Make sure your helper is holding your legs firmly against the table so you can fold your arms and hang comfortably (Figure 10.3).

You should feel no pressure on your pubic bone; rather, your weight should be borne on the upper thighbones. If you feel pain in the fronts of your thighs, use a blanket for padding. If you have tight hamstrings, bend your knees and have your helper secure you by pressing down on your thighs. If you are fortunate enough to have two helpers, the other one can tell you which side of your back is overstretched and which is collapsing so that you can begin learning subtle balancing adjustments.

To come out of the pose, place your hands on the floor below you and support your weight without moving your body while your helper comes around to steady the chair (Figure 10.4). Hold the chair seat and slide your legs close to the side of the table so you can put one leg down at a time.

Breathing and Imagery. Release your torso from the need to support itself. Relax your face and jaws. Inhale into your abdomen. On the exhalation, release your back. Continue to breathe and release. Let the heaviness of your head pull down on your spine. See your spine elongate. See your paraspinal muscles being stretched. See space being created between your vertebrae, allowing the discs to expand. See and feel your back becoming more symmetrical with each exhalation.

The gentle power of the breath can be used to help restore symmetry to your rib cage. Imagine a "crisscross" inhalation, in which you breathe into the front ribs on the side where the back ribs protrude and into the back ribs on the side where the front ribs protrude. For example, if your rib prominence is on the right side of your back, your right front ribs and your left back ribs will be "sunken in." Breathing into these sunken areas will help reduce the pain of collapse and stimulate your ribs to grow into a healthier alignment.

Cautions

- Be careful getting into and out of this position. Until you are quite secure with it, always have a friend help you, as you can strain your back and make things worse if you move incorrectly. Always get up slowly, holding on in case you should feel dizzy.
- This pose is a quick fix for many people with back pain, as the success of the many antigravity devices on the market indicates. And therein lies its danger: With quick relief from hanging, you may be inclined to stop with temporary pain relief and neglect postural reeducation. But used alone, hanging can actually lead, in the long run, to an unstable back. Stretching alone is insufficient: It must be accompanied by proper strengthening of the muscles that support your back and align your pelvis.
- This is an inversion. Therefore it should not be done by people with hypertension or a history of stroke, glaucoma, or diabetic retinopathy. It should not be practiced during menstrual bleeding.

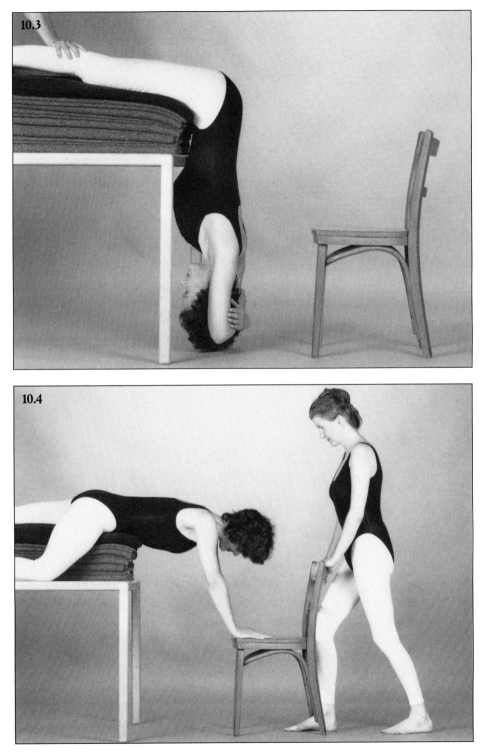

10.3   Hanging
10.4   Hanging, Exiting the Pose

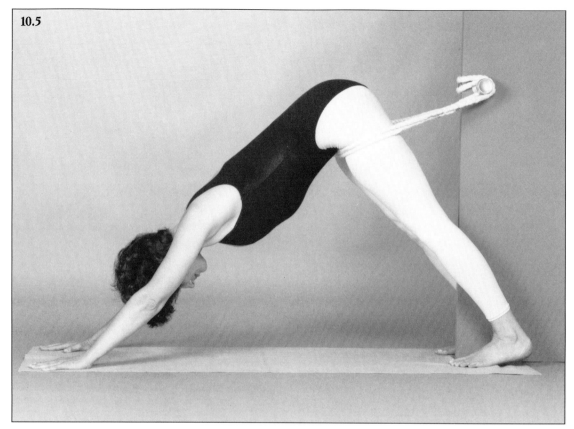

10.5

10.5   Downward-Facing Dog Pose, with Rope

Rationale. This pose reverses the effects of weight bearing and gravity on the discs and the facet joints. It stretches out the paraspinal muscles, thereby relieving spinal compression. It gives you the chance to recover from the destructive effects of collapse of the concavity and overstretch of the convexity, which are aggravated by gravity and fatigue. It is good to hang before practicing your yoga, so that you start out collapsed as little as possible.

Note

• *Do not practice this pose during the second half of pregnancy.*

Downward-Facing Dog Pose with Rope

Props needed: loop of soft cotton rope or cotton
strap, thick towel, door with sturdy doorknob.

Position and Adjustment. Make a loop of soft cotton rope or a cotton strap and hook it securely over both sides of a sturdy doorknob. Make sure that the doorknob is strong and secure enough to support your weight. Step into the loop and place it where your hips bend at the groin. Lean forward into the rope until your weight is supported and place your hands on the floor for stability and support as you walk your feet backward. Then walk your hands out in front of you to form the upside-down V of the pose (Figure 10.5). (Use a thick towel to pad the rope if it cuts into your hips.) If your hamstrings are too tight to do the pose with your hands on the floor, put your hands on the seat of a sturdy chair (Figure 7.34).

To increase symmetry in your spine, move one hand out farther on the floor than the other. Your helper can tell you which hand provides more spinal correction. Be sure not to let the shoulder blade on the side of the rib protuberance move toward the head. Keep both shoulders moving away from your ears. Hang for several minutes, keeping your legs activated by pressing your heels toward the floor.

Breathing and Imagery. Allow your spine to lengthen from your tailbone to the top of your head with each breath. Imagine roots growing from your palms, fingers, soles, and toes, pulling your hands and feet into the floor.

Rationale. This pose offers you a chance to recover from the painful effects of gravity-induced collapse. In addition, the support of the rope allows you to get a sense of where your lateral spinal curves are and to practice controlling them. In this pose, the helper can give advice by touching an area of concavity collapse and saying, "Stretch here, make more space," or touching an area of convexity overstretch and saying, "Decrease the amount of stretch you feel here. Take this part of your spine back toward the other side."

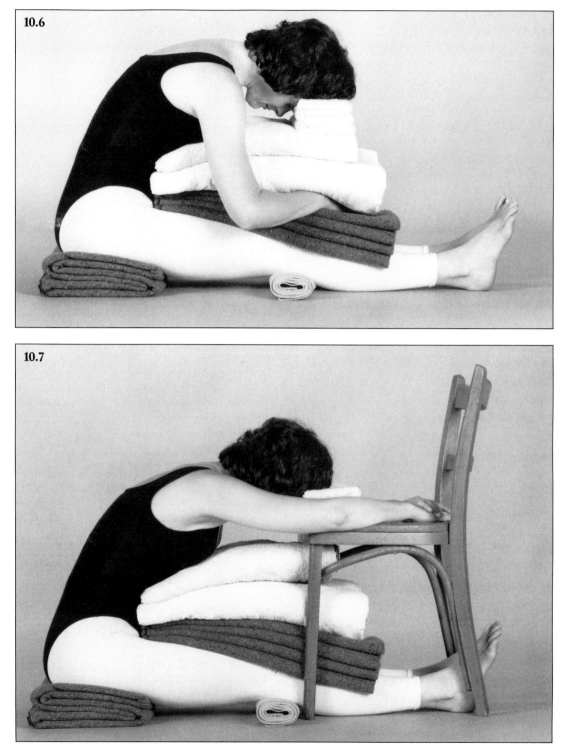

10.6   Forward Bend with Torso Support
10.7   Forward Bend with Torso and Head Support, for Limited Flexibility

✤
Forward Bend with Torso Support

Props needed: four to six folded blankets, padding.
(As needed: chair, necktie or cotton strap,
rolled towel.)

Position and Adjustment. Doing this pose safely requires adapting it to your flexibility. If the evaluation of your hamstring flexibility has shown that you have very flexible hamstrings, then you can do this pose seated on the floor. If your hamstrings are less flexible, this pose should be done while seated on several folded blankets at a height of four to ten inches. Place several folded blankets lengthwise on top of your legs and bend forward from your hips so your chest can rest on the blankets (Figure 10.6). Additional folded towels may be required under your head and neck, so your head can rest without a kink in your neck. If this is not comfortable, place a chair over your legs, put the blankets in your lap to support your ribs, and rest your head on the chair seat (Figure 10.7).

If your hands can easily reach your feet, hold your feet. If not, loop a necktie or cotton strap around your feet and hold that with each hand. Don't allow the shoulder blade on the side of the rib prominence to ride up, but keep it low on your back. If you are sitting on blankets, a rolled towel behind your knees will make the pose more comfortable.

Breathing and Imagery. Stay in the pose, using the Relaxation Breath (pausing at the end of each exhalation for several seconds before inhaling again). See your back elongating. Surrender your neck muscles and the weight of your head and your chest to the support of the props. Allow your spine to be supported from the front as you rest your chest on the blankets. Continually release the muscles at the base of your skull. Stay in the pose for thirty seconds to three minutes for the first several months. Then gradually increase the time to five to ten minutes by adding one minute per month.

Rationale. If the thoracic curve is abnormally flattened, this position encourages a more normal thoracic rounding. If the upper back is already rounded, the pose helps the upper back muscles release their tension so the spine can begin to lengthen. It allows the paraspinal muscles to stretch and lengthen in a relaxed and supported position.

Notes

- *If you have spondylolysis, spondylolisthesis, or posterior or lateral bulging discs, do not attempt this pose.*
- *Do not practice this pose during the second half of pregnancy.*

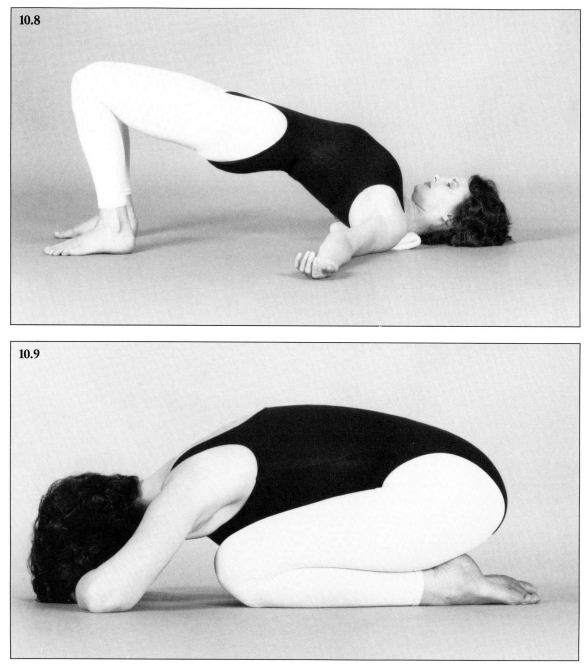

10.8   **Active Bridge Pose**
10.9   **Child's Pose**

Active Bridge Pose

Props needed: nonskid surface.

Position and Adjustment. Lie on your back on a nonslip surface, such as a hardwood floor or a nonskid mat. Bend your knees and place your feet parallel to each other, approximately six to twelve inches from your buttocks.

Inhale. As you exhale, press your feet, shoulders, and lower back firmly into the floor. Inhale again and, as you exhale, slowly begin lifting your spine from the floor, one vertebra at a time, beginning at the tailbone and proceeding upward toward the head (Figure 10.8). Keep your shoulders, face, eyes, and jaw relaxed and passive. Keep your thighs parallel. Do not allow your knees to fall away from each other.

During the entire exercise, keep your pubic bone moving strongly toward your breastbone.

Lift as much of your spine as possible off the floor. See if you can lift as far up as the middle to upper thoracic spine. Inhale, and on the next exhalation, slowly begin setting your spine back down on the floor, one vertebra at a time, beginning at the highest vertebra and proceeding downward toward the tailbone. Remember to keep your pubic bone moving in the direction of your breastbone and your buttocks sweeping down toward the backs of your knees. Repeat three to five times. Then rest in Child's Pose (Figure 10.9).

Pay special attention to the areas of the spine that seem to come down onto the floor in a block of several vertebrae, rather than one vertebra at a time. Work more slowly in these areas, so that vertebrae can move individually, both when you lift the spine and when you set it back down. It may be helpful to reach one hand under your back to touch each vertebra in turn as you set your spine down.

Do not be discouraged if you are able to lift your spine only an inch or two off the floor. Lifting any amount is beneficial.

Breathing and Imagery. Do not hold your breath. Move on a smooth exhalation, keeping your face relaxed. Imagine your spine as a string of large beads, each capable of moving independently of its neighbors. As you lift your spine into Active Bridge Pose, imagine that one end of the string of beads is being lifted slowly, so that each bead comes up in its turn. While coming back down, allow the string of beads to be set back on the floor one at a time, starting at the head and proceeding toward the sacrum.

Rationale. This pose teaches awareness of spinal movement while creating strength in the abdominal and back muscles, which support and move the spine. It also helps you to become aware of the connections among the shoulders, neck, and spine. You will quickly become aware of the shoulder and neck tension created by spinal movements. You will then learn to keep your shoulders and neck relaxed while your spine is moving independently of them. In scoliosis, especially the type in which the thoracic curve is flattened

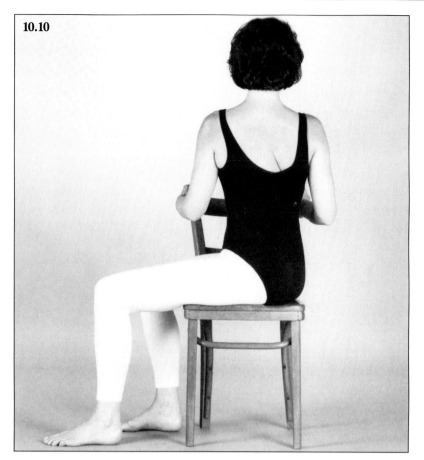

10.10

10.10 Seated Twist
10.11 Forward Triangle Pose

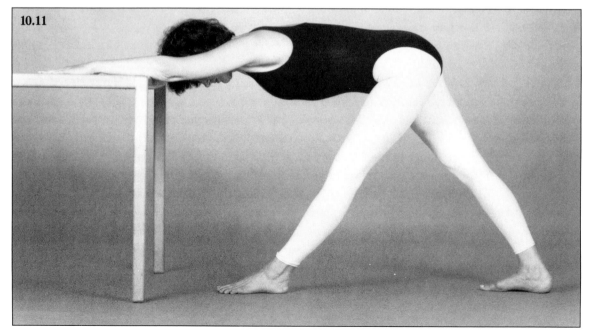

10.11

as well as rotated, the vertebrae can feel as if they are welded together. This pose releases the vertebrae from their bondage and teaches them to move more normally, as individual segments, rather than as a block.

Note

• *Do not practice this pose during the second half of pregnancy.*

❧

Seated Twist

Props needed: straight chair with flat seat.
(As needed: books, blanket.)

Position and Adjustment. Sit sideways in a straight-backed chair with a flat seat. Make sure that your feet are flat on the floor, with the ankles beneath the knees. If your feet do not reach the floor, place books under them. If your knees are higher than your hips, sit on a folded blanket high enough to raise your hips to the level of your knees. Be sure you are sitting on your sitting bones, not on your sacrum and tailbone. Place your hands on the chair back.

The twisting movement of this pose is coordinated with the breath. On one inhalation and exhalation, allow your spine to lengthen upward. Inhale, and on the next exhalation, gently twist your torso toward the back of the chair (Figure 10.10). Continue this coordinated breathing and rotation until you feel pain along the spine or ribs.

At this point your helper can give you advice by touching the painful area and telling you whether you are collapsing along the concavity (the inside edge of the side-to-side curvature) or overstretching a protruding area along the convexity (the outside edge of the curvature). With this information, undo the twist to the point just before the pain began. Then retrace the twist, but this time follow your helper's advice to avoid collapse or overstretch of the previously painful area. You will be surprised to see that you can now twist farther without pain.

Never try to twist past the point where pain begins. Always release the twist and try it again with new awareness in the area where the pain occurred. Once you attain your maximum pain-free twist, hold it for several breaths and then come out of the twist in the same way; slowly, moving on the exhalation, not allowing areas of convexity to overstretch or areas of concavity to collapse. Then repeat the twist with the other side toward the back of the chair. Remember to keep your shoulders low and relaxed. Repeat several sets.

Breathing and Imagery. Breathe smoothly and gently, using the Relaxation Breath. Visualize a "crisscross" inhalation that takes the air into the front ribs on the side where the back ribs are prominent and into the back ribs on the side where the front ribs are prominent. As you see your breath balancing the rib cage, visualize your spine growing longer and straighter with each inhalation. With each exhalation, maintain this new symmetry and length.

Rationale. This pose teaches the control you need to avoid pain due to collapse and overstretch. Patient teamwork with your helper will help you redefine what the word "straight" means.

❧

Forward Triangle Pose

Props needed: table, nonskid mat.

Position and Adjustment. Stand facing a table with your feet hip-width apart. Step one foot three to three and one-half feet behind the other. Make sure that your feet are parallel and your toes are pointing toward the table. (It's okay if the heel of the back foot does not touch the floor.) Activate your legs by pressing your heels downward. Inhale, and on an exhalation, allow your spine to lengthen upward. Inhale, and on the next exhalation, bend your torso forward at the hip joints (not at your waist), placing your outstretched hands on the table for support (Figure 10.11).

Stay in this position, breathing quietly, elongating your spine with each breath. To draw your attention to problem areas, your helper can lightly touch the concave side of your spine to remind you not to let it collapse, and the convex side to remind you to avoid overstretching. Make sure that your hips and pelvis are even, so one hip is not closer to the table than the other.

To come out of the pose, push down with your feet and strongly stretch out and up with your arms to bring your torso back to the standing position. If this feels too strenuous, press down on the table and use the strength of your arms to help you lift your trunk. Repeat on the other side. Do two to four sets.

Standing Poses

In addition to the poses described in this chapter, you should regularly practice the standing poses described in Chapter 7, "Moving On Poses." These poses are extremely important for people with scoliosis. Each standing pose helps balance muscular strength and length so that spinal symmetry can improve. Strengthening and coordinating all the major posture-determining muscle groups helps maintain the postural improvements.

Triangle Pose (Figure 7.5) and Revolved Triangle Pose (Figure 7.10) are especially important, because they balance out variations in the two sides of the body, especially important in scoliosis. They are also particularly good at strengthening the paraspinal muscles and the abdominal muscles. When the arms are used actively, these poses strengthen the upper back muscles, which stabilize the shoulder blades and help maintain an erect posture.

Arm Raises (Figures 9.6–9.7) also strengthen these muscles. This improved shoulder blade stabilization helps to reduce pain in the muscles and nerves around the shoulder blade on the side of the rib prominence.

While practicing the standing poses, beware of the tendency for the spine to collapse on the concavity and simultaneously overstretch on the convexity. The helper should give advice to prevent this from happening.

Some people believe that certain standing poses should be done only toward the side that creates more correction of the scoliosis. This is not true. There is plenty of work to be done on both sides when using the standing poses for scoliosis correction. No matter which side appears to give more correction, the same principles of normalizing the configuration of the spine apply: Never allow the concavity to collapse further, never continue to overstretch the convexity.

Rest Your Back

Always end your routine with one or two of the poses in Chapter 5, "Relaxation Techniques." Use additional padding, as necessary, to support the back on the side opposite the rib prominence.

Suggested Routines

Fifteen Minutes

1. Hanging, two minutes (Figure 10.3)
2. Downward-Facing Dog Pose with Rope, one minute (Figure 10.5)
3. Forward Bend with Torso Support, two minutes (Figures 10.6, 10.7)
4. Active Bridge Pose, three times (Figures 10.8, 10.9)
5. Triangle Pose, two sets (Figures 7.1–7.5)
6. Revolved Triangle Pose, two sets (Figures 7.7–7.10)
7. Forward Triangle Pose, two sets (Figure 10.11)
8. Child's Pose (or other Relaxation pose), remaining time (Figure 5.11)

Twenty Minutes

1. Hanging, two minutes (Figure 10.3)
2. Forward Bend with Torso Support, two minutes (Figures 10.6, 10.7)
3. Seated Twist, two sets (Figure 10.10)
4. Downward-Facing Dog Pose with Rope, one minute (Figure 10.5)
5. Active Bridge Pose, three times (Figures 10.8, 10.9)
6. Arm Raises, ten to fifteen times (Figures 9.6, 9.7)
7. Triangle Pose, two sets (Figures 7.1–7.5)
8. Revolved Triangle Pose, two sets (Figures 7.7–7.10)
9. Warrior Pose, two sets (Figures 7.16–7.18)
10. Child's Pose (or other Relaxation pose), remaining time (Figure 5.11)

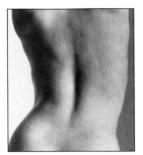

Eleven

A Woman's Back

Not only are women subject to the same back injuries that men are, but they are also at risk for back pain unique to those who have breasts, ovaries, and a uterus, who sometimes wear high-heeled shoes, and who experience the menstrual cycle, pregnancy, nursing, endometriosis, premenstrual syndrome (PMS), and postmenopausal osteoporosis.

Heavy breasts, lactation, nursing, and child care all encourage rounded shoulders, forward head carriage, and increased rounding of the upper back. The upper back muscles (especially the rhomboids, which connect the shoulder blades to the spine) can become painfully strained. In addition, lifting and holding children places an extra load on the lumbar discs. Exercises given in Chapter 9 for forward head, kyphosis, and neck pain are helpful. Also review the section on lifting in Chapter 12, "The Yoga of Daily Living."

PMS, Endometriosis, and Back Pain

Premenstrual syndrome (PMS) and endometriosis (displaced fragments of uterine lining) are both well-known female health challenges. The symptoms of PMS (including depression, mood swings, emotional fragility, fluid retention, food cravings, pelvic pain) and the pain and infertility caused by endometriosis are widely recognized. What is less well known, however, is that both of these conditions can be associated with back pain.

In two clinical studies of women with premenstrual syndrome, one-fourth to three-fourths of the women with PMS reported back pain that began with ovulation and ended with the onset of menstruation. The exact cause of back pain in PMS is not well understood, but it may be related to the release of hormones called prostaglandins shortly after ovulation. (These hormones are also responsible for the uterine muscle contractions that women experience as cramps.)

Pelvic congestion can also be a cause of back pain in the premenstrual part of the cycle. The blood vessels in the pelvis become swollen and engorged with blood as a result of the hormonal effects of ovulation. The associated swelling in the soft tissues of the pelvis causes back pain in many women.

Endometriosis is a condition in which small pieces of uterine lining tissue (endometrium) become attached to the outer surfaces of the uterus, ovaries, fallopian tubes, bladder, and intestines. They are subject to the same hormonal influences as normally located endometrium. As the monthly cycle progresses, the areas of endometriosis gradually increase in thickness, just as the uterine lining does. When it comes time for menstruation, they begin to break apart and bleed. Unlike the uterine lining, however, this tissue has no way to move out of the body. Over time, this recurrent hemorrhage causes the pelvic organs to become stuck together with adhesions and scar tissue.

Endometriotic implants on the network of nerves at the back of the pelvis can cause back pain. They have even been shown to cause classic symptoms previously thought to result only from a herniated intervertebral disc.

Although yoga exercises for PMS and endometriosis cannot cure either condition, they can relieve some of the muscle spasm that occurs due to pelvic nerve irritation, and some of the discomfort of pelvic congestion. Perhaps just as important, exercises and relaxation impart a sense of control and help reduce feelings of stress, anxiety, and depression.

The poses B.K.S. Iyengar recommends for discomfort related to the menstrual cycle demonstrate his three cardinal principles of therapeutic yoga: *spreading* (creating space for fresh blood to enter the organ), *soaking* (providing time and space for fresh blood to bathe and nourish the organ), and *squeezing* (removing used blood and fluid by pressure). This approach helps alleviate pain related to pelvic congestion.

Guidelines for Yoga Practice
During Menstruation

Yoga teaches balance: balance of the body in relation to gravity; balance of the mind between action and observation; and balance of the neuroendocrine system between activity and relaxation.

Through a regular yoga practice, you learn which poses are effective in reestablishing balance in various aspects of your existence. Certain poses in this ancient discipline are particularly useful to establish inner balance during menstruation. These poses ease menstrual cramps, heavy bleeding, pelvic discomfort, and the lower back pain sometimes associated with menses. They are also effective at smoothing out the emotional rough edges some women encounter at this time of their cycle.

Just as some poses are helpful at period time, other poses should be avoided. These guidelines are based on sound physiological knowledge and time-tested applications of yogic principles to women's special needs. Women are cyclic beings. For a woman to deny this fact interrupts the self-understanding she seeks through yoga.

The time of menstruation can be welcomed as a time for going within and allowing yourself to have low energy. Use this time to experience different aspects of your nature. High-energy exercise and vigorous yoga needs to be balanced by the quiet and peace gentle yoga can offer. The time of menstruation is a perfect time to vary your exercise routine by turning inward.

In general, poses requiring exertion and great energy are not recommended during the first few days of menstruation. Physical strength may be somewhat diminished at this time, causing you to be shaky or off balance. Attempting a strenuous practice when your energy is low can lead to injury or further depletion of energy supplies. This is a time to allow yourself to rest by practicing the restorative yoga poses that follow.

Yoga Poses for Back Pain with PMS, Menstruation, and Endometriosis

Wide Angle Pose

Props needed: folded blankets.
(As needed: two rolled towels.)

Position and Adjustment. Sit on a firm stack of neatly folded blankets with straight legs spread wide, facing a wall, with your feet touching the wall (Figure 11.1). Make sure that you are sitting firmly on your sitting bones. If your back rounds or your knees can't stay straight (Figure 11.2, Incorrect), sit on more blankets.

Your legs should be spread enough to stretch your inner thighs, but not to the point of pain. If your knees hurt, try putting a rolled towel behind each knee. Actively stretch your legs by pushing out with the heels and pulling back with the toes. From this base you can lengthen your spine. Keep your chin and shoulders low and your breastbone lifted. Use your hands pushing down behind your buttocks to help yourself sit erect and keep your breastbone lifted. Keep your legs active by stretching out through your heels. Stay here for one to three minutes, keeping your legs and torso active. Support your knees with your hands as you bend your legs to come out of the pose.

Breathing and Imagery. Focus on quiet breathing. See your pelvic floor widening and your spine lengthening upward.

Rationale. This spreading pose creates space in your pelvis to allow cleansing blood to enter and remove swelling and waste products.

Note

• *To use this pose in the second half of pregnancy, sit with your back to the wall and a fan-folded blanket behind your waist (Figure 11.3).*

❧

Reclining Cobbler's Pose with Chest Support

Props needed: folded blankets, head pad,
neck support roll, wall.

Position and Adjustment. Fold a firm blanket like a paper fan, so that it is approximately four to six inches wide, four to eight inches thick, and as long as the length of your body from just below your waist to the top of your head. Facing a wall, sit on the floor with the blanket behind you and pull it toward you so it touches your buttocks. Fold your legs in toward your body so the soles of your feet are touching each other and your toes are pressing against the wall. Using your arms for support, let your spine down onto the blanket. Use your neck support roll and head pad to support your head comfortably. Place your arms out to either side, with your palms facing up (Figure 11.4). If your inner thighs feel overstretched, either move your buttocks farther away from the wall, so there is more distance between your heels and your buttocks, or support each knee with folded blankets.

Breathing and Imagery. Rest in this position, using the Relaxation Breath, for thirty seconds to several minutes. Visualize softening the muscles around your hip joints and in your pelvis to release any tension brought on by back discomfort. This is an open, receptive pose. Sense the receptiveness of the whole body as your lungs receive each inhalation.

Rationale. This soaking pose allows cleansing, nourishing blood into your pelvis while stretching the inner thigh muscles.

❧

Reclining Kneeling Pose

Props needed: wooden block (or several books),
blankets, head pad, neck roll. (As needed: rolled
towel, folded towels, belt, socks.)

Position and Adjustment. This pose requires sufficient propping to support your trunk comfortably, while keeping your knees in contact with the floor and your thighs parallel. Even flexible students who could practice this pose without props should take advantage of the deep relaxation the props allow.

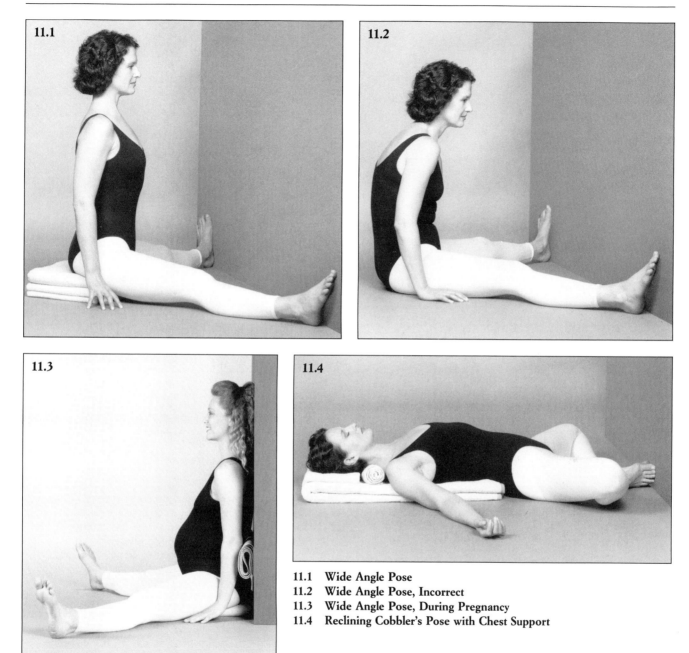

11.1   Wide Angle Pose
11.2   Wide Angle Pose, Incorrect
11.3   Wide Angle Pose, During Pregnancy
11.4   Reclining Cobbler's Pose with Chest Support

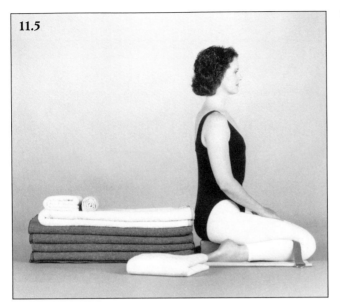

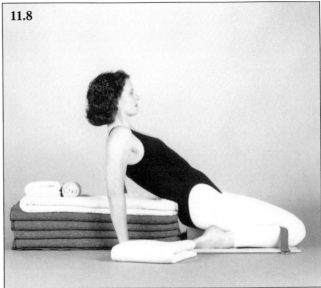

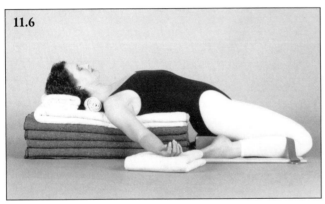

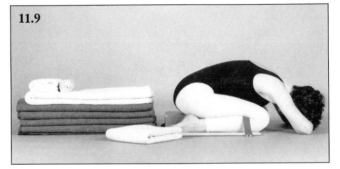

11.5 Reclining Kneeling Pose, Starting Position
11.6 Reclining Kneeling Pose
11.7 Reclining Kneeling Pose, Incorrect Head Position
11.8 Reclining Kneeling Pose, Exiting Pose
11.9 Reclining Kneeling Pose, Resting After

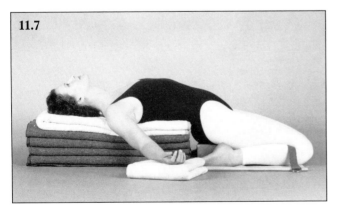

Kneel on a blanket with a ten- to fourteen-inch stack of fan-folded blankets behind you. (Yoga bolsters can also be used. See Resources.) Have your knees close together and your thighs parallel. Your head pad and neck support roll should be in place on the end of the blankets. Separate your feet and place a four-to six-inch wooden block (or a stack of books) between them to sit on (Figure 11.5). Using the strength of your hands pressing into the floor beside your buttocks, gently lower your trunk onto the blankets behind you.

Proper support for your head and neck is crucial for relaxation. (To refresh your memory about proper head and neck padding, refer to the detailed description in Chapter 5, "Relaxation Techniques," and see Figures 5.3–5.5.) You may need thicker padding than you do for lying flat (Figure 11.6). Adjust your padding so that your throat does not feel either stretched or compressed (Figure 11.7, Incorrect).

Reclining Kneeling Pose is best performed on a firm, noncompressible mat, such as a nonskid mat. You should not feel pain where your knees and tops of your feet come into contact with the floor. If you do, kneel on thicker padding. If the inside of the knee joint hurts, come out of the pose and insert a twisted sock into the crease of the knee before sitting on the block. If the ankles and tops of the feet hurt, place a rolled towel one to three inches thick under each ankle.

Do not allow your knees to separate widely. If they do, place a belt or strap in the bend of the knees before you sit down.

Knee joint or lower back pain calls for an increase in the height of the trunk or buttock supports. If your elbows do not reach the floor, put folded towels under your forearms for support.

To come out of the pose, move your trunk into an upright position by pushing your hands into the floor near your waist (Figure 11.8). Then, still kneeling, separate your knees and stretch your trunk forward. Rest your forehead on the floor or a folded blanket (Figure 11.9). Lengthen, relax, and release your back.

Breathing and Imagery. Stay in the pose thirty seconds at first, gradually building up to five minutes. Use the Relaxation Breath. See your body as a graceful arch extending from your knees to your shoulders. Visualize widening and lengthening from the pubic area to the navel.

Rationale. This squeezing and spreading pose reduces congestion in the pelvis and pacifies the nerves and muscles of the back and abdomen by increasing the space available for the pelvic and abdominal organs. Its chest-opening action also helps correct rounded upper back and shoulders.

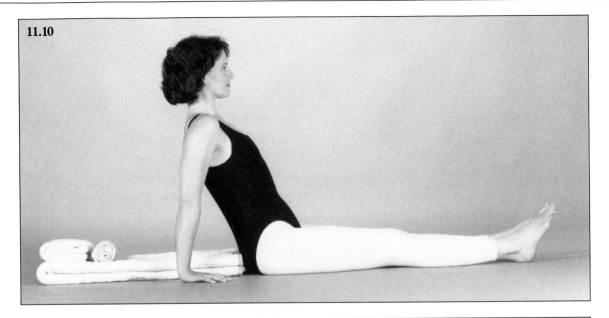

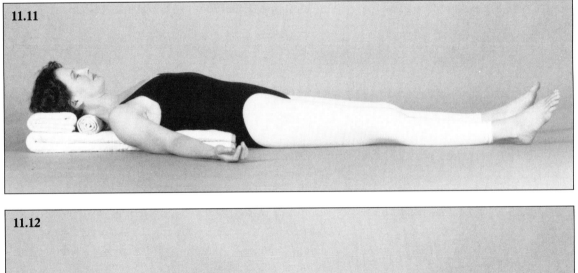

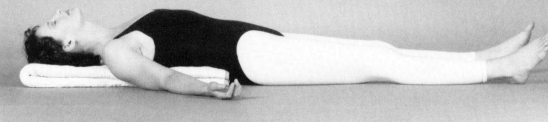

11.10 Supine Resting Pose with Chest Support, Starting Position
11.11 Supine Resting Pose with Chest Support
11.12 Supine Resting Pose with Chest Support, Incorrect Head Position

❦

Supine Resting Pose with Chest Support

Props needed: stack of two fanfolded blankets,
folded towel or blanket, rolled blanket,
head pad and neck support roll.

Position and Adjustment. Sit with your legs outstretched and a stack of folded blankets two to six inches high behind you, pressed against your sacrum. Using your arms for support, lean back onto the blankets (Figure 11.10). Support your head and neck with your head pad and neck support roll placed on top of the blankets (Figure 11.11). This support will keep you from hyperextending your neck (Figure 11.12, Incorrect). Rest in the pose for thirty seconds, gradually building up to five minutes.

If your lower back is uncomfortable, try one or more of the following maneuvers:

- Sweep your hands down under your buttocks toward your thighs to adjust the flesh and release your lumbar spine.
- Bend your knees. Press your feet to the floor and lift your buttocks. Lengthen the lumbar curve by moving your pubic bone toward your navel. Then set your hips back on the floor while keeping length in your lumbar spine.
- Lower the trunk support.
- Place a rolled blanket behind your knees.

As in the preceding poses, head and neck alignment is of utmost importance. Avoid throat compression or neck hyperextension by using adequate support under your neck and head. You may need thicker head and neck padding in this pose than when you are lying flat.

To come out of the pose, roll off the blankets onto one side, taking your head and neck padding along for a pillow. Rest there for several minutes, enjoying the feelings of deep and nurturing relaxation.

Breathing and Imagery. Breathe softly and gently, using the Relaxation Breath. With each inhalation, imagine that the breath is filling your entire torso and pelvis with cleansing air. With each exhalation, imagine that the breath is taking with it tension and waste products.

Rationale. In this pose, the supported opening of the rib cage facilitates deep relaxation. It soothes the nerves, allows for a deepening of the circulatory effects of the previous poses on pelvic congestion, and further releases irritated muscles.

Other Useful Poses

Practicing the standing poses described in Chapter 7 (using a table for support) can ease back pain during menstruation. Pelvic pain and congestion may cause the muscles in the pelvis to become tense, which may lead to back pain. Standing poses gently stretch and release these muscles. The Relaxation poses described in Chapter 5 are also useful, especially those that squeeze the abdomen, such as Child's Pose (Figure 5.11) and Supine Child's Pose (Figure 5.10). Also especially beneficial is Forward Bend with Torso Support (Figures 10.6 and 10.7). Visualize the squeezing action of these poses, seeing swelling leave the pelvis with every exhalation.

Back Pain with Pregnancy

Pregnancy puts your lower back at risk for mechanical strain in several ways. The enlarging uterus stretches the abdominal muscles, so they are no longer able to support the lumbar spine from the front. As pregnancy progresses, the center of gravity is moved forward from its usual place just behind the navel. This forward pull puts additional strain on the lumbar spine.

Back pain can also be caused by the enlarged uterus resting on the nerves at the base of the spine. And the hormone relaxin, produced during pregnancy to allow easier delivery, allows ligaments and tendons to stretch more easily. For these reasons, the usual muscular and ligamentous support of the back and other joints is reduced, and strains can easily occur.

If you are pregnant and considering a fitness program, begin by consulting your physician about the safety and appropriateness of the exercises under consideration. Some conditions that complicate pregnancy (hypertension, diabetes, toxemia, premature labor, and so on) can be made worse by some forms of exercise.

The guidelines for exercise during pregnancy are as follows:

- Never compress the abdomen or pelvis.
- Be sure to warm up before and cool down after exercising.
- Never allow breathing to become strained.
- Avoid bouncing or jarring activities.
- Avoid overstretching.
- Don't get tired.
- Remember that your center of gravity is shifting. Avoid activities in which you might lose your balance and fall.
- Be sure that your heart rate never exceeds one hundred forty beats per minute.
- Do not do inverted poses (such as Headstand and Shoulderstand) unless you are very experienced in them prior to pregnancy. Even then, get help from a teacher to lift your legs into these poses.
- Walking is excellent exercise during pregnancy. See Chapter 13, "Exercising Safely."

Yoga for Back Pain During Pregnancy

Constant postural awareness, especially while walking for exercise, will help to prevent back pain during pregnancy. Do not allow the weight of the baby and the uterus to increase the lumbar curve by tilting the pelvis forward and down.

After the fourth month, Side-Lying Relaxation (Figure 11.13) will help alleviate back pain. Lie on your side with a firm pillow supporting the head, a folded blanket supporting the belly, and another folded blanket under the top knee. In this position use the Relaxation Breath and visualize the lower back muscles lengthening. Also visualize the baby being nurtured by your healthy breathing and quiet relaxation.

Note

- *When you are lying on your back, the enlarging uterus can compress the vena cava (the huge vein at the back of the pelvis that drains the legs, pelvis, and abdomen, returning the blood to the heart). For this reason, avoid lying on your back during the second half of pregnancy. If you ever feel like you are going to faint while lying on your back, this is a sign of vena cava compression. Simply turn onto your side to get relief and remember not to do this again.*

Wall Squat

Props needed: chair, wall. (As needed: low stool or pile of books.)

Position and Adjustment. Stand with the wall at your back and your heels approximately eight to fourteen inches away from the wall, with your feet approximately one to one and one-half feet apart. Without leaning on the wall, squat, while keeping your knees wide enough to accommodate your baby. Hold a chair for support, if you need it. Then lean back on the wall to relax your back (Figure 11.14). Stay in this position thirty seconds to two minutes or as long as it feels good. You may be more comfortable sitting on a low stool or pile of books four to ten inches high (Figure 11.15).

Relax your face and jaw. Let your shoulders rest on the wall. If the back of your head does not rest comfortably on the wall, don't force it.

To come up, press your hands into the wall until your weight is over your toes and then press your palms firmly down onto your legs above your knees to help straighten your legs. Actively push down with your feet and lift up from the top of your head as you stand.

Breathing and Imagery. Use the Relaxation Breath. Feel your lower back lengthening with each inhalation and exhalation. Allow the support of the wall to help the muscles of your back release and lengthen.

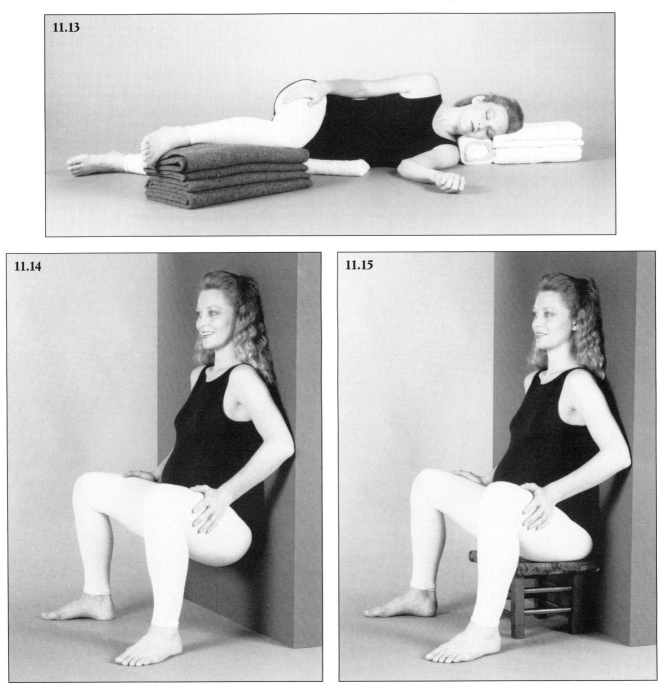

11.13 Side-Lying Relaxation, During Pregnancy
11.14 Wall Squat
11.15 Wall Squat, with Stool

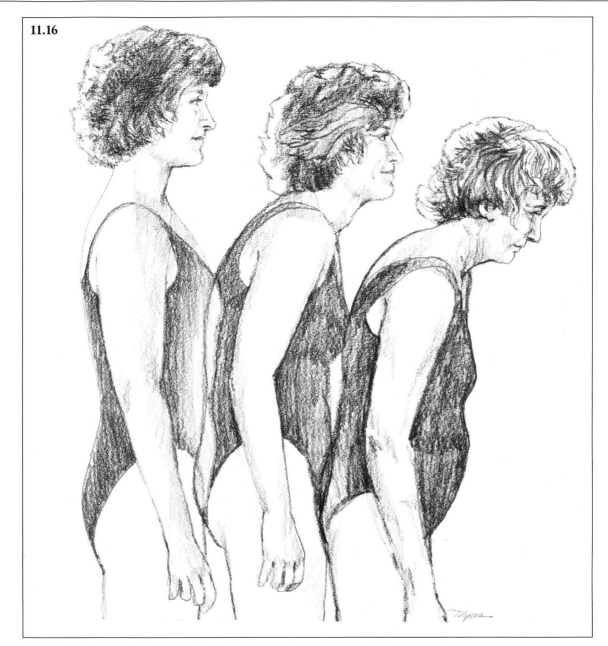

11.16 Vertebral Wedge Fractures Cause Progressive Loss of Height in Osteoporosis

Rationale. This pose eases backache by stretching the muscles alongside the spine in a supported position.

Use of the Home Base and Moving On
Poses During Pregnancy

Many of the Home Base and Moving On exercises in Chapters 6 and 7 are great for pregnancy. Check the "Notes" section of each pose description for tips on its use during pregnancy. When using these poses in pregnancy, never compress your growing baby. During the second half of pregnancy, eliminate any poses that require lying on your back. All of the poses in this book are excellent postpartum exercises.

Osteoporosis

Osteoporosis is a disease that causes the bones to become porous and vulnerable to fracture. Even a mild bump, stumble, or strain that the average person would barely notice can cause a bone to break if a person has osteoporosis. Vertebral, hip, and wrist fractures are characteristic of the disease, although osteoporotic persons can fracture any bone more easily than a normal person would.

Osteoporosis is really two separate diseases. One form of osteoporosis develops gradually with age in both women and men. In the other form, known as post-menopausal osteoporosis, insufficient estrogen production by the ovaries accelerates bone loss. This condition may occur naturally in menopause or prematurely when the ovaries are surgically removed. Excessive exercise or eating disorders such as anorexia nervosa or bulimia may also interfere with normal ovarian function.

Back Pain and Osteoporosis

Vertebral compression fractures occur most often in elderly men and in women within twenty years after menopause (if they have had no hormone replacement therapy). Pain in the midline over the spine results from muscle spasms associated with microscopic fractures of the collapsing vertebrae. Pain may be sudden and severe, or chronic and nagging. With repeated tiny fractures the vertebrae form wedges (narrow in front, wider behind), resulting in the dowager's hump (markedly increased thoracic curve) and loss of height (Figure 11.16). Vertebral fractures may occur after minimal bending and lifting. Neck, shoulder, and arm pain may develop because of altered spinal and shoulder mechanics. The lower ribs may even come to rest on the pelvic rim, collapsing the chest and interfering with breathing. As the diaphragm and the contents of the chest are pushed down, the abdominal organs protrude into a prominent belly. The resultant compression interferes with organ function. In addition, the neck and lower back become vulnerable to mechanical strain.

Exercise Cautions for Those with Osteoporosis

Be sure to avoid impact, sudden jerking movements, and any exercise that involves weight-bearing directly on the spine (for example, Headstand or Shoulderstand). Also avoid activities that reinforce a rounded back, such as rowing, or sit-ups or forward bends with poor alignment. Never tilt the head way back, as this action can compress the vertebral arteries.

Immediately after vertebral fractures, a back brace or corset may be necessary if any movement causes severe pain. In the long run, however, the benefits from a back brace must be weighed against the drawbacks of weakening the trunk muscles that support the spine.

Until vertebral fractures heal, practice gentle movements in a bathtub filled almost to the brim with water to provide buoyancy. Walk five minutes twice a day as soon as you can tolerate it. Increase the length of each walk by one minute each week until you are walking twenty minutes twice a day. Use the yoga of daily living (Chapter 12) while walking, sitting, and moving through your activities.

Swimming can increase mobility and muscle strength while the body is supported by the water. The buoyancy, however, makes swimming somewhat less effective than weight-bearing exercise, such as walking or yoga, at stimulating vertebrae to retain calcium. To strengthen the legs and hips, walk back and forth in the shallow end of the pool, using the pool edge for support, if necessary.

Yoga Poses for Osteoporosis

Exercises for the prevention of osteoporosis include weight-bearing exercises, such as walking and yoga. A forward head position and a somewhat rounded upper back usually precede the vertebral wedge fractures that cause dowager's hump. Correcting the forward head position early in life improves the biomechanical imbalances that can crush the anterior portions of the vertebrae. Chapter 9, "Rounded Upper Back, Forward Head Posture, and Neck Pain," addresses this type of postural correction. The Home Base and Moving On poses of Chapters 6 and 7 are also important in developing sufficient back and leg strength and flexibility to further protect the spine.

If you have recent or healing osteoporotic vertebral crush fractures, yoga poses should be limited to positions of comfort that provide spinal support while avoiding chest collapse and allowing for easy breathing (for example, Elbows on the Table, Figure 5.8; Side-Lying Relaxation, Figure 5.15; and Chair-Seated Forward Bend with Chest Support, Figure 11.17). Once vertebral fractures have healed, you can begin to select some of the poses in Chapters 5, 6, 7, and 9.

❧
Chair-Seated Forward Bend
with Chest Support

Props needed: two chairs, four to six blankets.
(As needed: thick towel.)

Position and Adjustment. Fold each blanket in half lengthwise, then fanfold it to create a rectangular support twelve inches wide. Roll the thick towel into a firm roll. Stack the blankets neatly and place them across the seat of one of the chairs, so that the long side of the stack is parallel with the back of the chair. (Yoga bolsters can also be used. See Resources.)

Sit in the other chair facing the side of the first chair. Spread your knees apart and pull the blanketed chair between your legs so that you are looking out over the long axis of the folded pile of blankets. Stretch your torso up as tall as is comfortably possible. Using your arms for support, lower your torso onto the pile of blankets. Place the rolled towel across your breastbone to support your upper chest. Allow your forehead to rest on the blankets or turn your head to one side and rest there for several minutes (Figure 11.17). Increase or decrease the thickness of the chest support by adding or taking away blankets until you are comfortable. To come up, use the support of your arms to push your torso back up to a seated position (Figure 11.18).

Breathing and Imagery. Use the Relaxation Breath. Feel your back ribs expand with each inhalation. Pause briefly at the end of each exhalation to allow further spontaneous release of the breath. See the muscles of your back relaxing and releasing tightness and spasm. See your vertebrae healing and becoming strong once again. See pain leaving your spine and your spine becoming longer with every exhalation.

Rationale. This pose offers the possibility of a few moments of comfort and easier breathing. Carefully adjust the thickness of the props until comfort is achieved. Although this is a forward bend, undue pressure is not placed on the anterior portions of the vertebrae because the spine is fully supported. With the abdomen relaxed, the back muscles can relax as well, thus freeing the back ribs for easier breathing.

Note

• *If you have posterior or lateral bulging discs, do not attempt this pose.*

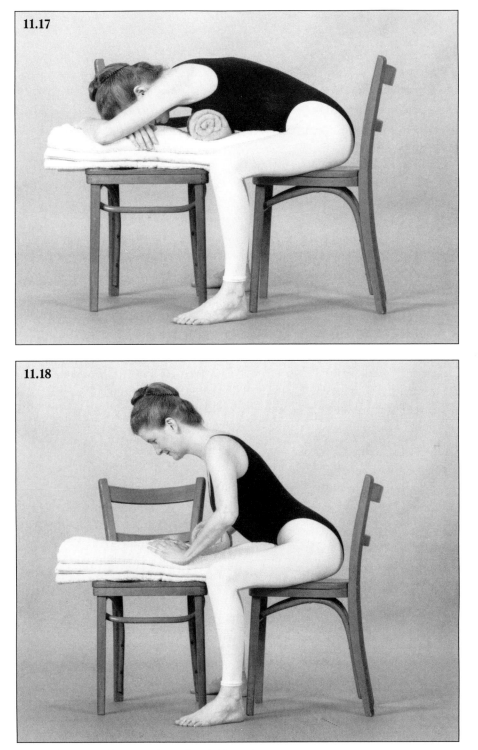

11.17 Chair-Seated Forward Bend with Torso Support
11.18 Chair-Seated Forward Bend with Torso Support, Exiting the Pose

Suggested Routines

For PMS, Endometriosis, and Menstrual Difficulties (fifteen minutes)

1. Child's Pose, two minutes (Figure 5.11)
2. Forward Bend with Torso Support, three minutes (Figures 10.6, 10.7)
3. Reclining Cobbler's Pose with Chest Support, three minutes (Figure 11.4)
4. Reclining Kneeling Pose, three minutes (Figures 11.6, 11.9)
5. Supine Resting Pose with Chest Support, two or more minutes (Figure 11.11)

(Optional additions for added back relief: Triangle Pose, Figure 7.4; and Revolved Triangle Pose, Figure 7.10. These poses can be inserted between Child's Pose and Forward Bend with Torso Support.)

For Osteoporosis

If you can tolerate them, practice the routines for kyphosis at the end of Chapter 9. If these are painful, practice only Chair-Seated Forward Bend with Chest Support (Figure 11.17), Elbows on the Table (Figure 5.8), and Side-Lying Relaxation (Figure 5.15).

During Pregnancy

During the first half of pregnancy, you can practice any of the Relaxation, Home Base, or Moving On routines described in Chapters 5, 6, and 7, while observing the precautions noted in this chapter.

During the second half of pregnancy, try the following fifteen-minute routine.

1. Wall Squat, one minute (Figure 11.14)
2. Wide Angle Pose, two minutes (Figure 11.3)
3. Kneeling Lunge, two minutes (Figures 6.16, 6.17)
4. Wall Push or Downward-Facing Dog Pose with a chair, one minute (Figures 7.25, 7.28, 7.34)
5. Triangle Pose, two sets (Figures 7.1–7.5)
6. Revolved Triangle Pose, two sets (Figures 7.7–7.10)
7. Warrior Pose, two sets (Figures 7.16–7.18)
8. Wall Push or Downward-Facing Dog Pose with a chair, one minute (Figures 7.25, 7.28, 7.34)
9. Side-Lying Relaxation, two minutes or longer (Figure 11.13)

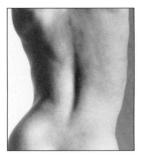

Twelve
The Yoga of Daily Living

*I*f your back is prone to pain, just getting through your daily activities can be like tip-toeing through a mine field. Almost any activity (and even inactivity) can cause problems if you don't practice proper body mechanics or if your strength or flexibility is insufficient.

If the new posture, inner awareness, and self-image that you are developing through your yoga practice disappear when your exercises are finished, your old habits will be constantly working against you the rest of the day. The lessons in this chapter will help you change destructive habits of movement and posture that can continually reinjure your back.

The process of transferring your newly developing sense of postural alignment to your everyday activities is a wonderful opportunity for self-exploration. To live in harmony with your back, consider all of your daily activities as an informal yoga practice.

The following are a few rules to move by in the yoga of everyday life.

Breathing Break and Posture Check

Whenever you can, take a few seconds for a breathing break and posture check. Take a long, slow inhalation into your abdomen and back. As you consciously exhale, check and adjust your posture. Let yourself feel taller and more erect (without lifting your chin). Relax your jaw and shoulders.

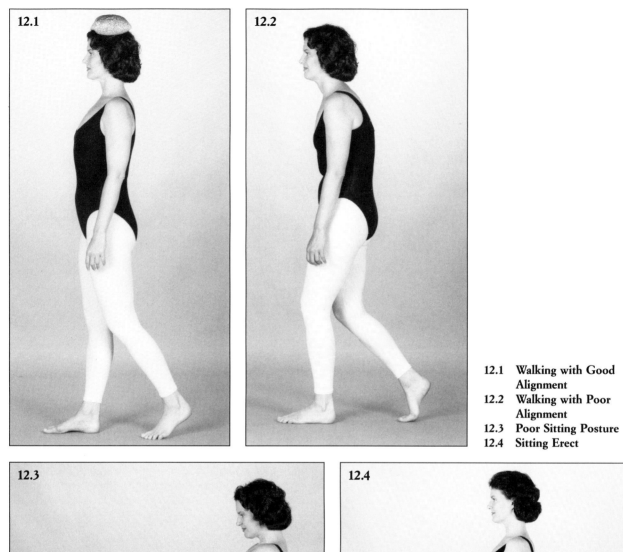

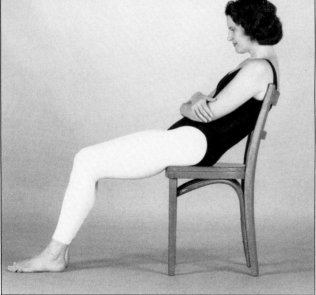

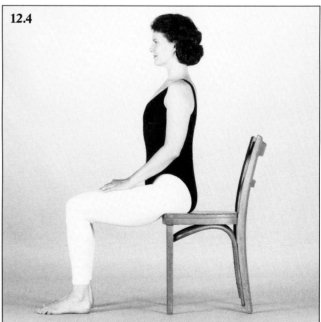

12.1 Walking with Good
      Alignment
12.2 Walking with Poor
      Alignment
12.3 Poor Sitting Posture
12.4 Sitting Erect

Standing and Walking

Move consciously and deliberately, mindful of how your body position affects your balance. Be aware of your center of gravity. When you are standing upright in correct alignment, your center of gravity lies behind your navel, and your weight is evenly distributed along the length of your spine.

When your center of gravity is chronically forward of your navel (because you stand with your shoulders stooped or your head forward or because you have a large, protruding belly), pressure is put too much on the front part of the vertebrae, rather than being evenly distributed over the entire vertebral surface. This uneven weight distribution increases the likelihood of back problems.

Stand and walk in Mountain Pose (Figure 6.22). Don't lean over or walk in a stooped, hunched posture. Avoid holding your arms crossed in front of your chest. Instead, try standing with them crossed behind your back, each hand holding the opposite elbow. Practice walking with a bag of rice or dried beans on your head (Figure 12.1). Feel as if your head is constantly pushing the weight up away from your ears. As much as possible, keep your ears over your shoulders, your shoulders over your hips, and your hips over your knees and feet. Let the top of your head, not your chin, reach upward. Don't lead with your chin (Figure 12.2, Incorrect). For more information about walking for exercise, see Chapter 13, "Exercising Safely."

Sitting

Sitting is particularly difficult for people with disc disease, as it increases the compressive forces on the lumbar vertebrae. Therefore, sit as little as possible. If you must sit, take breaks. Get up and move around frequently.

Sit on your sitting bones, not on your sacrum or tailbone. Sitting on your sacrum or tailbone flattens the lumbar curve and stresses the supporting muscles and ligaments (Figure 12.3, Incorrect). If your feet don't reach the floor, support them with a book.

Sitting erect. Sit on the front half of a firm flat chair seat with your head over your shoulders and your shoulders over your hips (Figure 12.4). This alignment strengthens the upper back muscles for better posture. Practice sitting in this position at least several minutes every day.

Sitting to read or watch television. Use an armchair with a high, firm back. Place a firmly rolled towel behind your waist to support your lumbar curve. (Once you've determined the proper thickness, use tape or rubber bands to secure the roll.) Pin or tape another rolled towel to the chair behind your neck and a folded towel behind your head for additional support.

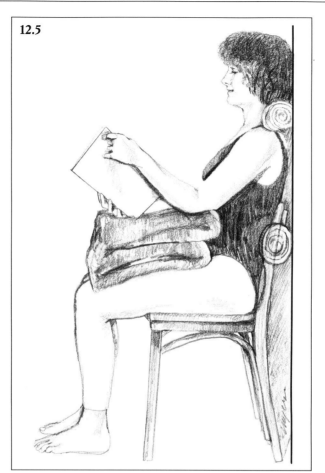

12.5   Sitting To Read
12.6   Getting Up from a Chair

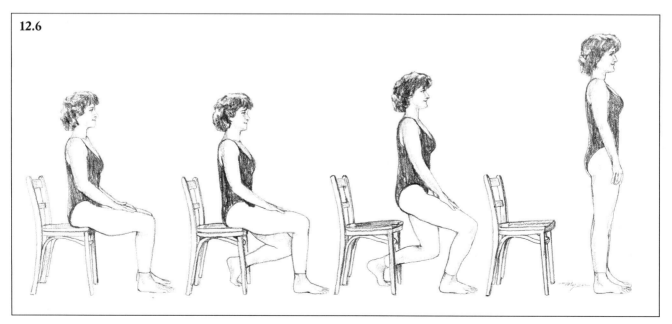

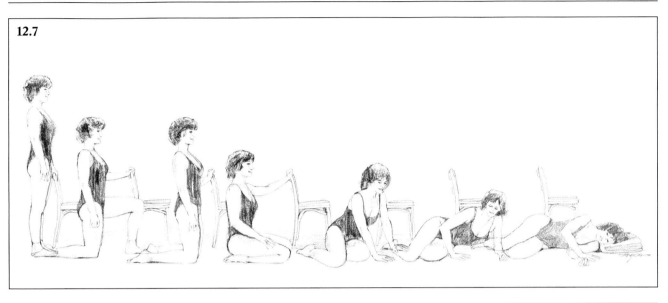

12.7

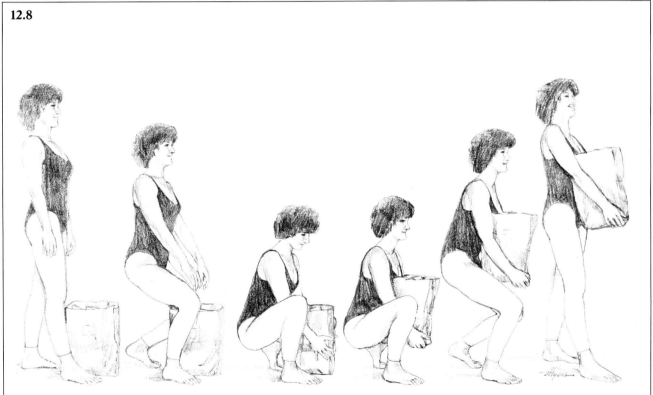

12.8

12.7   Getting Down To and Up From the Floor
12.8   Lifting

To read in this position, elevate your book so you don't have to hang your head forward to read (Figure 12.5). Prop your forearms and the bottom of the book on a support resting on your lap, such as a piece of firm foam rubber, a pillow, or a box. Keep these props handy so you'll remember to use them.

Getting up from a chair. Avoid low, soft chairs. Whenever possible, choose a firm chair with arms whose seat surface is level with the bend of the back of your knee. When getting up, don't lead with your chin. Keep your head aligned over your center of gravity. Move to the edge of the chair seat. If possible, place one foot under the chair seat, with the other slightly forward. If this is not possible, turn your knees, feet, and body to one side. Let your entire trunk and head lean forward as a unit until your center of gravity is over your feet. Then push down with your hands and feet to stand (Figure 12.6).

Reverse the process to sit down. Don't lean your torso forward and lead with your buttocks. Instead, stand close to the chair, with one foot partially under the chair seat, if possible. Lower your erect body straight down onto the edge of the seat. Then slide back into the chair.

Getting down to and up from the floor. Practice this at least once a day. Poor body mechanics while getting up and down can stress your lower back, while correct movement protects and strengthens it. If you practice getting up and down with good body mechanics, that way of moving becomes a new good habit. The correct action becomes engrained so that when you practice your yoga poses on the floor—or sit on the floor for any other reason—you will automatically get up and down in a safe manner.

From a standing position, firmly place one foot slightly behind the other. Using a sturdy piece of furniture as needed for support, go down on one knee, keeping your ears over your center of gravity. Then kneel on both knees. Take your buttocks back toward your heels and sit to the side of your feet. To lie down, use your arms to ease one side of the trunk down to the floor (Figure 12.7). To stand, reverse this process. This is how you should always get into and out of any yoga poses practiced on the floor.

Lifting

The farther away from the body you hold an object, the more pressure is put on your vertebrae. (For every pound held one foot from the front of the body at waist level, fifteen pounds of pressure are transferred to the lumbar discs: Holding a twenty-pound child or grocery bag transmits a whopping three hundred-pound load to the spine!) The closer you hold an object to your body, the more evenly its weight is distributed over the length of your spine, pelvis, and legs. And because your center of gravity is shifted only minimally, you are less likely to lose your balance and fall.

Get as close as possible to the object, then go down on one knee. Hug the load to your abdomen while lifting with the strength of the legs (Figure 12.8). Straighten your legs by pushing down firmly with both feet. Do not overdo. Get help if you need it. Divide a large load into several smaller ones. Never stand or squat to the side of your object—this position would require you to lift and twist at the same time, an action that can shred the outer rings of the intervertebral discs. (To understand how twisting can injure the outer layers of a disc, visualize wringing out a mop. The inner strands of the mop are twisted very little, while the outer strands, which have farther to go, receive more of the torque, or twisting force.) *Never lean over or bend from the waist to pick up anything.* Always bend your knees to get your body down to the proper level. If you find that you must lean over for some reason, support part of your body weight by pressing one hand down onto your thigh or a sturdy piece of furniture.

Lifting and carrying babies and children. It may take some ingenuity to apply the yoga of daily living to child care. Purchase or modify beds and playpens so you are not required to lean over to lift the child out. Set up a place to change diapers where you can stand erect or kneel. It is far better to carry the child on your back than on your hip or attached to the front of your chest. Carrying your baby in a plastic infant seat with a handle causes back strain because it forces you to hold the weight farther from your center of gravity.

Sleeping

Remember to get enough sleep to give your discs a chance to soak up healing nutrients. Sleep on your back with a pillow behind your knees to release the lumbar vertebrae from the pull of the hip flexor muscles (Figure 12.9). If you wish to sleep on your side, bend at your hips and knees. Elongate the waist on your down side by increasing the distance from the hip to the armpit. Do this by moving the hip away from the armpit. Placing a pillow between your knees, or under the knee of the top leg, may feel good (Figure 12.10). And, of course, use a firm mattress.

Experiment with lumbar support for sleep. Fanfold a long towel, wrap it comfortably around your waist, and secure it with a safety pin. It will stay in place no matter how much you toss and turn. Try different thicknesses and placements. Some people like it best at waist level, but others find that it works better lower on the hips.

Unless you have a tight piriformis or flat lumbar curve, avoid sleeping on your stomach. This position can strain the lumbar discs.

If you are a stomach sleeper by habit, begin to change your sleep position by starting off lying on your side or back. Relax in this position for a while before you turn over to sleep. Gradually, over many months, you'll find that you'll learn to go to sleep in one of the new positions. Be patient.

Some find waterbeds comfortable, others don't. If you do use a waterbed, make sure it is full enough to provide adequate support. The newer "baffled" waterbeds provide more support than the old single bag ones.

Before you get up, stretch in bed. Pull your knees to your chest for a little while, then roll onto your side and get up.

Driving

Position the seat back so it is as erect as possible. You may get more back support with the seat closer to the steering wheel. Adjust your driving seat with folded or rolled towels so you are sitting on your sitting bones with your lower back supported. To give yourself more support and to keep from slumping, fold a bath towel in half and roll it into a firm, tight roll. Secure it with tape or rubber bands. Place it lengthwise down your spine, above your sacrum. Alternatively, roll a hand or bath towel (depending on the thickness desired) and place it crosswise (perpendicular to the spine) behind your waist to provide lumbar support. See which works best for your back and your car seat. You may like to keep both handy so you can alternate on a long trip.

Commercially available foam rubber lumbar rolls and driving pillows are usually less effective at providing back support than are firmly rolled towels adjusted exactly for your own back. Compressible foam is too soft to support the bones, and the amount of support gradually decreases as the pillow flattens. The larger back pillows for driving are designed for the average person and may not fit your back and your car seat at all.

Experiment with towels of different lengths and thicknesses held in place by tape or rubber bands. When you find what works, secure the shape with more tape. Keep these posture props in the car, so they'll always be with you when you need them. On long airplane trips, similar props can be fashioned from the airline sleeping pillows and blankets. Don't be shy. Ask for what you need to be comfortable.

On long drives, take breaks every few hours. Do some of the easy stretches from Chapter 7, such as Wall Push (Figure 7.25). At a rest area, do Supine Pelvic Tilt (Figure 6.1) and Sacral Rock I and II (Figures 8.2, 8.3) while lying on a picnic table.

Getting in and out of a car. Open the car door and stand with your back to the door opening, facing away from the car. Place one hand on the back of the car seat and the other on the steering wheel or dashboard for support as you gently lower yourself down into the seat, leaving your legs on the outside of the car.

Using your hands for support on the steering wheel, dashboard, or car seat, rotate your entire body as one unit to bring yourself into a forward-facing position with both legs in the car.

To get out of the car, reverse the process. First open the door. Then use your arms to rotate your entire body as a unit so that your legs are outside the car. Finally, slide your buttocks toward the edge of the car seat and use the strength of your arms to help you push up into a standing position.

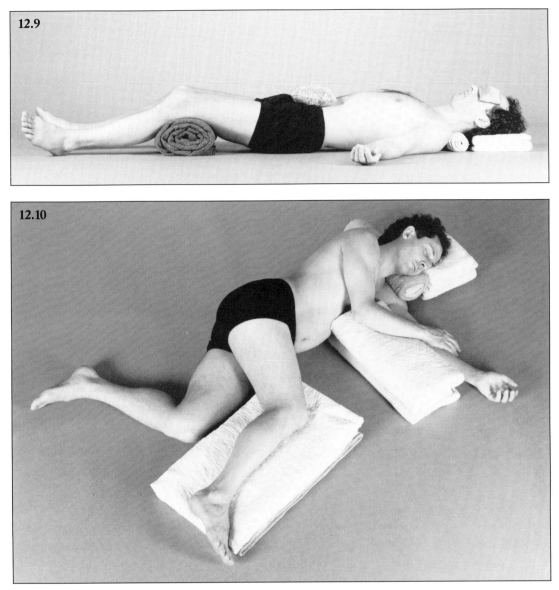

12.9   **Supine Resting Pose with Knee Support**
12.10 **Side-Lying Relaxation**

Be especially careful with the lifting and twisting actions required to put a child in a safety restraint seat. As soon as possible, teach the child to climb into the seat unassisted.

Housework

Spread out the load. Involve other members of the family in household chores. If you live alone, spread the household chores out over several hours, days, or weeks. Help yourself by decreasing the amount of tracked-in dirt: Begin a family tradition of removing shoes at the front door, a custom in Asia and in Hawaii.

Vacuuming. Vacuuming is a chore that easily lends itself to being done in small increments. Vacuum the house one room at a time over several days. Keep your body erect and don't lean over the vacuum wand. Make sure the wand is long enough that you can stand up straight. Let the vacuum do the work; don't press the suction device into the carpet. If you have a thick pile carpet, consider using a vacuum with a separate electric motor on the floor attachment. Hold the vacuum pipe or the handle of an upright unit close to your hips. Alternate hands and the sides of the body on which you hold the machine. Use good body mechanics when manipulating the heavy parts of the machine. Don't yank on the hose to reposition the machine; rather, walk back to it and squat or kneel to reposition it.

Sweeping. Hold the broom close to your body and stand erect, using the full length of the broom, rather than leaning over toward the floor. Alternate the hand that is on top and the side of the body you hold the broom.

Watering houseplants. If you have many plants, divide this chore over several days. Carry small amounts of water at a time, if necessary. Use a watering can with a long spout. Try to arrange plants so you don't have to lean over to water them.

Ironing. Avoid ironing by beginning to add to your wardrobe clothes that don't require it. Consider this a long-term partial solution to the problem. Break up ironing into small batches. Have each family member iron his or her own clothes from as early an age as is safely possible. Stand erect. Avoid leaning over the ironing board. It may be comfortable to rest one foot on a small stool. Alternate feet and avoid leaning into the hip of the standing leg.

Washing dishes. This is another chore that can be shared with other members of the household. Have one person do the cooking, another the clean-up. If possible, clean up during the preparation phase as well as after the meal, to break up the time spent standing at the sink. If you have a dishwasher, have each family member rinse and load his or her own dishes. Cook in or on foil, when possible, to avoid hard-to-clean, baked-on food. Good tools, such as scrubbing sponges and firm brushes, help. While doing these chores, stand in Mountain Pose (Figure 6.22).

Making the bed and changing bed linens. Don't lean over the bed—work one side at a time. Kneel at the side of the bed on one or both knees. In order to get close to the bed while on one knee, turn slightly to one side. Put a pad between the knee and the floor for comfort. Remember that if your hip flexor muscles are short, kneeling on both knees at the same time may cause overarching of your lumbar spine and lead to strain.

Grooming

Brushing your teeth, washing your face, and shaving. Stand erect. Don't lean over the sink. It may be helpful to place another mirror on a wall away from the sink so that you can get close to it without leaning over. To wash your face, use a washcloth, rather than leaning over to splash water from the sink. Avoid sticking your head forward and your chin out. Try using an electric shaver while standing in Mountain Pose (Figure 6.22). If you must get closer to the mirror to see adequately, lean on one arm.

Washing your hair. Use a shower, if at all possible. Don't lean over the sink or crouch in the tub to put your head under the faucet. When shampooing in the shower, don't allow your lumbar spine to overarch when you raise your arms.

Yardwork

Gardening. Get as much help with gardening as you can. Consider decreasing your gardening ambitions to match the stamina of your back. Garden in small increments, alternating the more vigorous leaning and bending chores with easier tasks. Do not sit on the ground with your back rounded. Instead, sit on a stool, or wear knee pads and kneel. Check gardening supply catalogues for aids such as gardening stools and knee pads. Be careful when lifting. Never lift and twist simultaneously.

Digging and shoveling. Avoid digging and shoveling until your back has been free of pain for at least six to eight months, and your yoga program has progressed into the Moving On poses in Chapter 7. Even then, start small: small amounts of time and small loads on the shovel. Keep the loaded shovel close to your body. Shoveling fresh, loose snow or loose soil is much easier than wet, hard-packed snow or earth. Bend at the knees, not the back, to lower the shovel. Do poses from Chapter 5, "Relaxation Techniques," before and after any heavy yardwork.

Construction Work

Be very careful with body mechanics during lifting. Remember that your lower back is at risk when your arms are raised overhead (as in nailing or painting). Stand on a ladder or scaffolding to avoid reaching overhead.

Office Work

Sitting places markedly increased pressure on the lumbar discs. Therefore, your chair is very important. A kneeling chair (such as a Balans, where the seat is slanted forward and the body weight is on the sitting bones and the shins) is fine for keeping the spine erect in tasks that require you to lean forward slightly or be erect (such as microscope work or sewing). For tasks in which you usually lean back slightly, you need a chair with an adjustable back and an adjustable lumbar support. Make sure that the chair seat is of the proper height, so your feet can rest flat on the floor, with your knees and hips bent at ninety degrees. The lumbar support should be adjusted specifically for *your* back. If other people use the chair, make sure that you readjust it when your work begins. A variety of chairs and tools are available to help with correct, comfortable posture (see Resources).

Arrange your work surface and work materials at a proper height. Have your computer screen at eye level so you don't have to look up or down. Place the keyboard so you don't have to lift your shoulders in order to rest your hands comfortably on the keyboard.

Avoid holding the telephone receiver in place by squeezing it between your shoulder and your neck. Alternate ears. Use a headset, if possible. Speaker phones, for hands-off use, are great.

Try a stand-up desk, or use an elevated surface, such as the top of a file cabinet. There is less pressure on the lumbar discs while standing than while sitting.

Sexual Intercourse

A back injury, unfortunately, may lead to deterioration in your sex life. Beginning as a fear of reinjury, this can lead to alienation from your mate, which can lead to depression, which can, in turn, lead to even further alienation.

Just as your yoga program can offer an opportunity to explore and develop new ways of moving in exercises, so this program can offer new skills for enhancing the quality of your most intimate relationships and for continuing to enjoy sexual intercourse despite a back injury. Partners can approach lovemaking positively, even therapeutically, rather than allowing the emotions of fear and alienation to prevail. Work together to provide enough time and a relaxed environment for gentle, playful exploration. Here are a few suggestions:

- Use some foreplay time to do resting poses and gentle stretches together, perhaps to soothing, gentle music.
- Use peaceful, gentle, slow, and controlled movements, not frantic thrusting, jerking, or twisting movements. This pace can be facilitated with appropriate music.
- The safer intercourse positions allow the partner with the injury to be less active and more supported by the firm mattress surface and pillows. Keeping the knees bent helps protect the lower back. If sleeping with a towel pinned around your waist has been helpful, try that for lumbar support during intercourse as well. Avoid flattening or overarching your lumbar curve. Experiment to find comfortable positions that are just right for you and your partner. See Resources for an excellent booklet on sex and back pain.
- Remember that proper alignment is just as important in the bedroom as anywhere else. Stay attuned to signals that you might be stressing your back, and adjust your posture and positions accordingly.
- Consider methods of achieving orgasm other than vaginal intercourse.
- When your lovemaking is over, don't forget to rest and realign yourself with one or two Relaxation poses such as Lying Down with Calves on a Chair (Figure 5.7) or Supine Child's Pose (Figure 5.10).

Take this rebuilding of a healthy sex life as an opportunity to explore and improve your relationship. As you develop better communication and accommodate each other's needs, your relationship will increase in strength and flexibility, just as your body does.

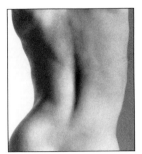

Thirteen

Exercising Safely

"When will I be able to dance again?"

"I don't feel good about myself when I'm not able to run. Can you help me improve my back so that I'll be able to run again?"

"I get more enjoyment out of playing golf than almost anything else in my life. Please don't tell me I'll never be able to do it again."

Quite often someone with back pain comes to me with the specific purpose of improving back health in order to be able once again to enjoy a favorite sport that causes back difficulties. My response varies from person to person, according to the extent and duration of the injury, the types of stresses the particular form of exercise places on the back, and the person's dedication to following a rehabilitative yoga program.

One person may be able to resume the activity with slight modifications and temporary decreases in intensity, duration, and frequency.

Someone else may need to discontinue the activity and work on back reconstruction with yoga. After a period of rebuilding, the activity may be tried again for short periods of time. If this trial period goes well, the sport can be resumed. If not, more back-building yoga is needed before another trial.

Yet another will realize that this favorite activity is always going to be problematic. Expectations must be adjusted to allow enjoyment of new activities instead.

This chapter points out potential causes of back injury in a number of sports and exercise techniques. It shows how to minimize chances for injury by altering your approach and describes specific strength and flexibility preparations. And it outlines safe, enjoyable alternatives to injurious sports.

Aerobic Exercise

By now most people are familiar with the benefits of regular aerobic exercise for the heart, the circulatory system, and general well-being. Many recovering back patients have felt they were automatically excluded from aerobic exercise. However, there are a number of enjoyable aerobic exercises that can be beneficial for the back and require fewer precautions than most. These include walking, cross-country skiing, Nordic-type ski machines, low-impact aerobic dance, rowing and cycling with good posture, and swimming. Participating in these activities safely requires incorporating them into a rehabilitative yoga program that includes constant attention to alignment. All can provide an aerobic workout, with its salutary effects on your heart, state of mind, and metabolism.

Precautions for Aerobics

Precaution 1. Cardiovascular examination. Before you embark on an aerobic training program, you should have a thorough medical cardiovascular examination, including a stress electrocardiogram if you are older than thirty-five or have a family history of cardiovascular problems.

Precaution 2. Assess your postural alignment (as described in Chapter 4). Are you flat-footed, knock-kneed, bowlegged? Do you walk toed in or toed out? Are you swaybacked or is your lumbar curve flattened? Do you walk or run with your head set forward? If you are significantly out of line in any area, the repetitive action of running, walking, or dancing may cause problems for you in the joints affected by the misalignment. Use your yoga practice to help restore balance and proper alignment to these areas as you slowly begin to explore aerobic activity. If joint pains or lower back problems develop, decrease your level of aerobic activity until the symptoms abate. Proceed more slowly and concentrate on your yoga for a while. Give yourself time to adjust and improve your alignment before pushing ahead with an aerobics program.

Precaution 3. Stretch before and after aerobic exercise. Stretches for warming up and cooling down are a vital part of a complete aerobics program. Here yoga practitioners have an advantage over those who understand little about proper stretching. Most aerobic endeavors use the same muscle groups over and over. If these muscles are not stretched *before* a workout, they can tear. If they are not stretched *after* a workout, they will become progressively shorter, pulling the pelvis out of proper alignment, preventing full mobility of the joints, and placing the back at risk. Home Base and Moving On stretches to prevent these problems are described in Chapters 6 and 7. Use them faithfully before and after aerobic exercise.

Precaution 4. Avoid aggressiveness and competitiveness. Your mental approach to aerobics is the key to stimulating, rather than irritating, the heart. If you approach such activities with an aggressive or competitive attitude, a full-blown stress response is likely to result. In contrast, when conducted introspectively, in a setting of safety and control, aerobics can be made less stressful while its stimulating and invigorating qualities are retained.

Approach your aerobics program with the yogic attitude of nonaggression and nonviolence toward yourself. It took you many years to get in the condition you're in now; now give yourself time to get back in shape. Start where you are and proceed at a pace dictated by your own abilities. Avoid trying to start where you think you should be. Free yourself from the tyranny of a chart in some book. Go at your own speed, listening to your body's messages and responses.

What are some of the signs that might indicate that your aerobic exercise is becoming irritating, rather than stimulating? While exercising you should feel none of the following: heart flutter or palpitations; irregular pulse; cold, clammy skin; nausea; anxiety; chest, neck, or arm pain; shortness of breath; or a feeling of impending doom. Afterwards you should feel no edginess or irritability. You may feel tired, perhaps; wiped out, no.

If you have any of the preceding symptoms or if you find yourself dreading your workout, consider the cause. Are you working harder than you're really ready to work? Do you have a physical problem that has gone unrecognized? Do you need to find another form of exercise? Listen to your body and your mind. Honor your own good sense. Keep adjusting your program until it is one you can look forward to and thoroughly enjoy. If you are unable to do this, consider medical reevaluation.

Walk Your Back to Health

Walking is great aerobic exercise, easily accessible to the person who has had back injury or surgery. I strongly recommend it to all who come to me for back therapy, once they are over the acute pain and no longer have frequent muscle spasms. It is a wonderful, positive substitute when other forms of aerobic exercise cause back problems.

Here are some of the benefits of walking for the back:

- Walking offers an excellent cardiovascular workout that can be fine-tuned to serve your needs from the early postinjury or postoperative period well into the years after a full recovery.
- Walking is a low-impact aerobic activity. Impact activities such as jogging and aerobic dancing are difficult for those with vulnerable lower backs. The impact of the feet hitting the ground or floor is transmitted up the skeleton and can place excessive stresses on the injured area. Any skeletal misalignments are greatly magnified by the momentum generated in high-impact aerobics.

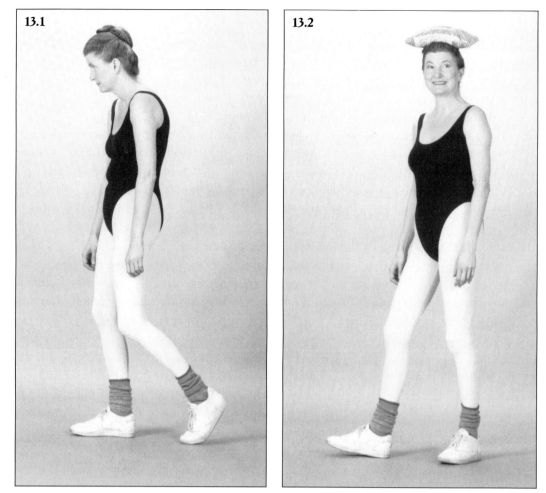

13.1   Walking with Poor Alignment
13.2   Walking with Good Alignment

- Walking provides the tranquilizing effect of moderate rhythmic exercise. The activation of major muscle groups can increase endorphin levels for pain relief without drugs.
- Walking provides you with an excellent opportunity to practice your new posture and body alignment skills.
- Walking helps strengthen all of the muscle groups that stabilize and protect your back.
- The easy swaying motion of the spine while walking provides circulatory benefits to the muscles, bones, and intervertebral discs.
- The psychological benefit of walking in spacious surroundings is enormous. In good weather you can be outdoors. In bad weather shopping malls are ideal. With every step you say to yourself in body language: I am doing something good for myself. I am helping my back become stronger and healthier. I am increasing my ability to tolerate pain. I am decreasing my tendency to cause myself pain.

The requirements for healthy walking are as follows: Good shoes. Even walking surface. Good company. Good attitude. Good posture. Good environment.

Walking is highly accessible. It does not require investment in a health club membership or in new clothes. It does not require lessons. The only equipment required is a good pair of walking shoes, which are useful for many other activities. An active walker will need new shoes about every six months. Stay on relatively flat, paved paths or sidewalks until you have built up your strength over six to ten months. Walking on uneven ground makes it hard to maintain good alignment. Hills are also difficult until you are strong and well aligned.

How To Walk for a Healthier Back

The best posture for healthy walking encourages the natural spinal curves. The head, chest, and pelvis are carried over the weight-bearing structures of the body (the hips, the legs, and the lumbar spine). When viewed from the side, a healthy walker will have the ears over the shoulders and the shoulders over the hips. In contrast to posture where the entire body is slanted forward or where the head is forward of the shoulders, this alignment allows the weight of your body to be properly balanced and avoids overworking the muscles of your back. When your body is slanted forward or part of it is forward of your center of gravity, your back muscles must overwork to keep you from falling over on your face (Figure 13.1).

Lightly activating the abdominal muscles supports the lumbar spine and aligns the pelvis. To activate your abdominal muscles, imagine your pubic bone moving up toward your navel. *Do not try to walk with so much abdominal muscle tension that you tuck your tailbone under and flatten your lumbar curve.*

While walking, do not try to hold your spine rigid, but allow it to have a sinuous motion from front to back in response to the movements of the legs. Imagine that the top of your head is moving up rather than forward as you walk. Imagine being suspended by a helium balloon from this spot. This allows your body to assume more natural spinal curves, with the ears in a more normal position over the shoulders. Imagining this spot lifting also keeps you from leading with your chin. Practice walking with a bag of beans on the top of your head, letting your head push up against the weight (Figure 13.2).

Drop your shoulders away from your ears. Release the muscles of the shoulders and upper back as much as possible without allowing your shoulders to slump forward. However, don't rigidly pull your shoulders back. Lightly lift your breastbone without over-arching your lumbar spine.

Let your arms swing naturally at your sides. (Don't exaggerate the arm swing as is done in racewalking.) Don't allow either arm to cross your midline, as this action can put excessive twisting forces on your lumbar spine and pelvis. Let your hands be relaxed. Make sure they are not clenched in fists. Suspend keys and other items on your belt so your hands can be free.

Let your stride be easy and natural. Don't try to artificially increase the length of your stride in an effort to work harder, as this can place undue strain on your back. Become aware of the direction your feet are pointing. Are they pointing straight ahead or out to either side? If the feet are not pointing straight ahead as you walk, do not change their direction immediately, which might put strain on your knees. Gradually, over time, allow your foot placement to change as your foot, knee, and leg alignment improves through therapeutic yoga.

Let your face muscles relax. Make sure that your jaw is not clenched. Your breathing should be gentle and even. If your breathing is so labored that you are unable to carry on a conversation or sing, then you are exerting too much effort. Slow down or switch to flat terrain.

Keeping an image in mind while walking can help improve walking posture effortlessly. Here are a few of my favorites. Try these, but don't hesitate to try out some of your own as well.

Be your own walking partner. Imagine that you are walking beside yourself, observing your posture from the side. As your observing self looks at your walking self, you see that your ears are directly over your shoulders, your shoulders are over your hips, and your spinal curves are nicely aligned. Your head and shoulders are not forward of your center of gravity. Watch yourself moving smoothly and efficiently. See how relaxed and healthy you look. Give yourself a smile.

Mirror yourself. Imagine that the surface you are walking on is a mirror. As you move along, feel the upward push of the feet of your reflection giving a lightness and buoyancy to your stride. Feel your own spine and head elongate toward the heavens just as the spine and head of your mirror image are drawn equally toward the center of the Earth.

Imagine that you are wearing a crown. Walk regally, not with your spine crushed down and compressed by the weight of the crown, but rather with your head and spine lifting the crown as if it were weightless. Do not lead with your chin, but keep the chin low and the back of your neck long. Allow yourself to feel noble. Smile at all you survey!

Low-Impact Sports and Exercises

Low-impact sports, such as rowing, cycling, cross-country skiing and the use of ski machines, and low-impact aerobic dancing, can be helpful for back rehabilitation, but can also be problematic in a number of situations. If these sports or activities are practiced with poor posture or poor alignment of the body with the equipment, your lower back can suffer.

Rowing and cycling are especially injurious if practiced with a rounded back or forward head. (Never row or cycle if your back pain is due to spondylolysis or spondylo-listhesis.) If rowing and cycling are practiced with good spinal alignment, injury is unlikely to occur. The newer trail bikes or all-terrain bikes allow better posture than do racing cycles. Cycling is notorious for strengthening and shortening the muscles at the front of the thigh (the hip flexors). Since these muscles pull on the front of the lumbar spine and pelvis, tightening them can cause the lower back to overarch. Make cycling safer by combining it with an erect cycling posture and by stretching the quadriceps and hip flexors before and after riding. Kneeling Lunge (Figures 6.16, 6.17) and Easy Bridge Pose (Figures 6.12, 6.13) are ideal to stretch these muscles.

Cross-country skiing and the use of ski machines require constant attention to keeping normal spinal curves with the head over the shoulders and the shoulders over the hips. The body should not lean forward more than five degrees. The shoulders should not be rounded or hunched.

Bench aerobics, stair climbing, and stair-climbing machines should all be performed with special attention to good posture. As your knees bend, make sure they move straight out over your toes; don't let your knees collapse toward the midline.

If you have a sensitive lower back, low-impact aerobic dancing can cause you problems if you lift your arms above your head. Remember that raising your arms can increase the curve in your lower back, especially if you have tight shoulders.

High-Impact Sports and Exercises

High-impact sports, such as running, jogging, dance, minitrampoline, gymnastics, and high-impact aerobics, can be dangerous if you are rebuilding your back. Momentum and speed decrease your ability to control posture and body mechanics. High-impact activities

activities send shocks through the body on each landing. Shock-absorbing ability is decreased if you have postural flaws involving the feet, knees, or spine, if you have soft tissue scarring, or if you have a degenerative joint disease, such as arthritis or bone spurs. In addition, the hip flexors and hamstrings are repeatedly shortened. The body can be pulled out of alignment unless these muscles are conscientiously stretched before and after exercise.

As a temporary solution, if you are a runner, jogger, or minitrampoline user, switch to walking (not racewalking) for the time being. If you are a dancer, change to ballroom dance or low-impact aerobic dance while your yoga program proceeds.

Later on, you can try small doses of your favorite high-impact sport or activity as part of a program that includes stretching, therapeutic yoga, and walking. See how it goes. If the addition of the high-impact sport or activity causes no problems, then you can safely continue. If a setback occurs, however, omit the offending activity for a few more months, continue to rebuild, and try again later.

If gymnastics-related back pain is due to spondylolysis or spondylolisthesis, it is best to explore other pleasurable forms of exercise. Continuing with acrobatics with either of these two conditions is not wise.

Fans of high-impact sports or activities can also try a mixture of aerobic activities that includes walking, swimming with mask and snorkel, low-impact aerobics, and the use of bicycle and ski machines with good posture.

Weights for Walking and Running

Do not wear weights on your hands or ankles during back rehabilitation. Wearing weights on the ankles while walking or running can cause problems in the feet, ankles, knees, hips, or lower back. The added weight only magnifies the detrimental effect of any misalignments.

Hand-held weights or weights wrapped around the wrists can also create problems. Because these weights are usually carried forward of the midline of the body, they shift the center of gravity forward, putting a considerable extra load on the lumbar spine and overworking the muscles in the lower back and neck. (Remember, the lumbar discs will feel the amount of weight that is held one foot in front of the navel magnified fifteen times.) Hand-held weights can increase problems if you have carpal tunnel syndrome (a repetitive motion injury of the wrists that causes the tissues of the wrists to swell and push on the nerve, causing weakness or numbness), as they exacerbate the muscle imbalances related to this condition. They also strengthen the front chest muscles, accentuating rounded shoulders and upper back. And if you have arthritis in the hands, elbows, or shoulders, using these weights may make it worse.

Swimming

Although swimming is excellent exercise if you have back challenges, it can still cause some problems. The lower back is in danger during the crawl, butterfly, back and breast strokes. As the arms are stretched forward and overhead, the curve of the lower back can be exaggerated. Also, lifting the head to breathe can irritate the neck.

Swimming can be changed into a totally positive rehabilitative back activity through the use of a mask and snorkel for the crawl and breast strokes: You can swim with your body aligned as in the Mountain Pose. If you choose not to use a mask and snorkel, turn your head to alternate sides for breathing. The side stroke is excellent for those with back challenges, but you must learn to alternate sides. (This may sound easier than it really is. I thought I would drown before I got the hang of the side stroke on my "wrong" side!) Don't neglect back strokes, but be careful not to overarch your lower back. Do the same number of back stroke laps as forward stroke laps. A swimming program should be accompanied by a program of stretching and strengthening exercises from Chapters 6 and 7, both before and after each swim.

Martial Arts

You must have excellent strength, alignment, posture, balance, and flexibility in order to practice the martial arts safely. If the martial arts are of great interest to you, use the Home Base and Moving On poses to prepare. The movements in judo, karate, tae-kwon-do, and other such arts require leg and hip strength and flexibility. The abrupt punching actions can torque the lumbar spine. Kicks can stress the lumbar spine if the legs and hips are not flexible enough for the legs to be lifted and extended while maintaining normal spinal curves.

In order to practice a martial art safely, you may need to spend a number of months practicing the standing poses in Chapter 7. Then begin slowly with only one martial arts class a week, making sure to do your therapeutic yoga daily, especially before and after class.

Bowling

Leaning forward *and* twisting *and* throwing a heavy bowling ball combines a number of potentially harmful actions for the lower back. Avoid bowling until you have been practicing rehabilitative yoga at least eight to twelve months and have been pain free for at least four months. Should you then wish to resume this sport, begin with a light ball and, for the first month, play no longer than fifteen to thirty minutes, no more than twice a week. If your back does not complain, slowly increase the amount of time you play. Definitely do not bowl if you have spondylolysis or spondylolisthesis.

Basketball

Playing basketball safely and well requires excellent strength, stability, alignment, and flexibility. The lower back is placed at risk many times each game. When the arms are raised for blocking and shooting, the lumbar curve may be exaggerated, which can cause injury. The quick turns and stop-start action require great leg strength, stability, and flexibility. The jarring impact of landing after jumping can cause problems if you have limited flexibility or less-than-perfect alignment. Finally, the rapid pace of basketball makes it almost impossible to pay constant attention to your alignment.

Clearly, if you have just sustained a back injury or undergone back surgery, basketball must wait. Use this interim time for building a better, stronger back using this book. Once you have been pain free for several months and are enjoying a regular, vigorous walking routine, you can begin to cautiously explore basketball again. Select teammates with abilities similar to your own. Start with playing only a few minutes on a half-court after a good session of warm-up stretches and exercises. Use your yoga exercises for warming up and cooling down.

Downhill Skiing

Safe skiing requires considerable strength and flexibility in the ankles, knees, and hips. There must be sufficient flexibility of the buttock muscles and hamstrings that you avoid skiing in a flat lumbar position. You must be able to rotate your upper spine as well as your lumbar spine in order to avoid lumbar strain. If your upper back, pelvis, or hips can't rotate freely, excessive rotation can be required of your lower back.

To ski more safely, work on leg strength, foot and knee alignment, leg and hip flexibility, and rotational flexibility of the upper back. The standing poses and spinal twists in Chapter 7 will be particularly beneficial.

Racket Sports, Golf, Baseball, Softball, and Other Asymmetric Activities

In addition to requiring leg and hip strength and flexibility, these sports use the body asymmetrically and require rotational movements that place heavy demands on the spine, pelvis, and sacroiliac joints. The asymmetrical use of the upper body, combined with rotation and the jarring impact of the swings, place the lumbar spine in danger if the hips, shoulders, and thoracic spine are tight. You risk developing pelvic misalignment and sacroiliac strain due to repeatedly twisting the pelvis to the same side. (Asymmetrical activities such as painting, working as a potter's wheel, and playing a stringed instrument place the same sort of rotational demands on the body.)

If you are a devotee of an asymmetric sport or activity, it is important to work on upper body flexibility. Remember that when the thoracic spine cannot rotate, the lumbar spine and pelvis must make up the difference. Thus you should use your yoga routine to gain flexibility and strength in your shoulders, hips, upper back, and legs. You should also work on improving the alignment of your head and neck: If you play an asymmetric sport with your upper back rounded or your head forward, you will not be able to rotate your upper body easily. Work with the poses in Chapter 9. You can also try alternating sides during practice sessions, playing with the opposite hand from the one you usually play with.

To speed your return to playing your asymmetric sport, practice standing poses and spinal twists (Chapter 7). Remember to stretch before and after each game. Remember always to bend at the knees when picking up the ball. Never lean over!

Weight Training

Weight lifting or weight training should not be attempted until you have progressed beyond the rehabilitative poses in this book and are able to participate in a regular yoga class without pain. Even then, any weight-lifting activity should be attempted only under the guidance of an exercise therapist or physical therapist. (Unfortunately, some of these professionals are not attuned enough to alignment to protect you from injury, so pay attention to your new sense of correct body mechanics. One of my back patients is an exercise therapist who perpetuated her back problem with poorly aligned use of weight-lifting machines.)

Working with weight-lifting machines can strengthen and enlarge muscles, but it doesn't teach coordinated total body movement or reeducate your postural habits as yoga does. Furthermore, weight lifting is often approached aggressively, with arbitrary numbers of repetitions and arbitrary weight goals in mind. This approach is inappropriate for back recovery, as it tempts you to overdo in seeking to attain a particular quantity rather than quality of movement.

Without a conscientious effort at postural improvement, weight training can actually reinforce poor postural habits and cause further misalignment. The strong muscles keep on doing most of the work while the weak muscles are allowed to stay lazy.

The bottom line about weight-training activities for back rehabilitation is this: As a solitary approach they are woefully inadequate and potentially harmful. They should be used only with the careful guidance of an exercise therapist or physical therapist (choose one who used to have a back problem) and then only as a part of a complete program that includes postural reeducation, intelligent stretching and strengthening exercise that teaches total body coordination (such as the yoga taught in this book) and therapeutic rest.

Note

• *You can get many of the strengthening effects of weight training through yoga, by lifting parts of your body—for example, by holding up the weight of the body, legs, and arms in the Moving On poses.)*

Abdominal Strengtheners

Athletic sit-ups with bent knees or with straight legs. Back patients often tell me, "I have done thousands of sit-ups, and my back has only gotten worse and my abdomen has gotten no flatter." Sit-ups are, all too often, incorrectly practiced with numerous repetitions by back patients and bodybuilders seeking an increase in abdominal muscle strength. In recent years, it has been learned that athletic sit-ups performed with the legs straight can hurt the back. As a result, sit-ups are now usually performed with bent knees. Unfortunately, people still try to come up into a complete sitting position. Just bending the knees is not enough to protect your back. Instead, you must modify the sit-up further, so that you lift only the head and shoulders off the floor. Don't go all the way to a full sitting position.

A review of the action of the muscles involved will help you understand how sit-ups should be performed if you are to increase abdominal strength without placing your lumbar spine at risk. In the action of sitting up from a straight-leg or bent-knee position, the abdominal muscles are responsible for lifting the trunk only thirty degrees or so off of the floor. (Slinging the arms forward uses the latissimus dorsi muscles—which go from the upper arm to the midback—to partially lift the trunk, letting the abdominals get by with less work.) After that the iliopsoas muscles (the main muscles that bend the thighs at the hips) lift the trunk up into the sitting position by pulling the lumbar vertebrae and lumbar discs away from the floor and toward the thighs. This pulling on the tissues of intervertebral discs and lumbar vertebrae can be quite destructive if your lower back is already vulnerable.

For safe abdominal strengthening, Yoga Sit-Ups (Figures 6.2–6.4) and Supine Knee-Chest Twist (Figures 6.5, 6.6) strengthen the abdominal muscles without putting the lower back at risk.

Supine leg raises. Lying on the back and lifting both straight legs is another so-called abdominal strengthener that is hard on the lower back. It requires the hip flexors to lift both legs at the same time. As the legs are lifted, the lower back is usually also lifted from the floor. If your abdominal muscles and hip flexor muscles are strong enough for you to lift the legs without lifting the lower back from the floor, this exercise can be performed with relative safety. For most people, however, especially those with lower back difficulties, this is not the case.

For safety, keep one knee bent with the foot flat on the floor. Then raise the other leg while keeping the lumbar spine pressed into the floor.

Stretching

Incorrect stretching, as I observe it being practiced on athletic fields and in parks and gyms, can be very harmful. Athletes need to be taught how to stretch safely, so they can obtain the benefits of back pain prevention and postural correction without injury.

Bouncing while stretching may seem like it helps you stretch farther, but it is actually counterproductive and can be injurious. Bouncing stretches lead to many of the injuries seen in aerobics classes. Your weight and momentum during bouncing can cause more stretch than your tissues can actually accommodate. This can result in microscopic tears of muscles, fascia, and tendons, which heal by scarring, further shortening the muscles and limiting flexibility.

Bouncing also activates the stretch reflex. (This is the reflex your doctor checks by tapping on the tendon just below the kneecap, causing your foot to kick.) Quickly stretching a muscle tendon (by tapping or by bouncing) causes the muscle to perceive that it is going to be overstretched. Its response is to contract and shorten its resting length. Therefore, bouncing stretches actually cause you to get tighter and tighter.

For safe stretches a position of mild to moderate stretch must be held in good alignment for at least fifteen to thirty seconds in order for the muscles to receive the physiological signal to lengthen. Therapeutic yoga stretching, or other stretching following the yogic principles of nonagression and attention to alignment, is the best way to lengthen muscles. The Home Base and Moving On poses provide excellent stretches for all sports.

Dear Reader,

      Now it's up to you. You have what I've given to each of my patients: a prescription for recovery tailored precisely for your body, your activities, and your goals. This book is a map showing you the way. With it, you can write your own prescription for a healthier back—including yoga for postural correction, pain relief and stress management; the yoga of daily living; and safe aerobic exercise. These are the fundamental components of a new approach to happy, productive living that should serve you well for years to come.

      I wish you all the best. You can do it!

      Sincerely,

      Mary Pullig Schatz, M.D.

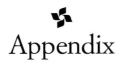

Appendix

Goal Diary

Date	Goal	Date Goal Achieved

Goal Diary

Date	Goal	Date Goal Achieved

Back Care Diary

Date	Circumstances/Causes of Back Attack	Pain Duration	Location & Severity (Mild/Moderate/Extreme)	Comments

Back Care Diary

Date	Circumstances/Causes of Back Attack	Pain Duration	Location & Severity (Mild/Moderate/Extreme)	Comments

Flexibility and Alignment Worksheet

	Date ☞		
Seated Evaluation of Lumbar Curve (Figures 4.1–4.3) flat, normal, sway			
Standing Evaluation of Lumbar Curve (Figures 4.4–4.6) flat, normal, sway			
Evaluation of Thoracic Curve (Figures 4.7–4.8) increased, normal, decreased			
Evaluation of Right Shoulder Roundedness and Right Shoulder Blade Position (Figures 4.9–4.11) rounded, normal, high, low			
Evaluation of Left Shoulder Roundedness and Left Shoulder Blade Position (Figures 4.9–4.11) rounded, normal, high, low			

Evaluation of Standing Alignment from Side (Figure 4.12)
    Head
    forward, normal, back			

Center of Knee Joint (right) behind ankle, over ankle, in front of ankle			
Center of Knee Joint (left) behind ankle, over ankle, in front of ankle			
Evaluation of Standing Alignment from Back (Figures 4.13, 4.14) spine straight, lateral curves			

Evaluation for Possible Scoliosis (Figure 4.15)
    back ribs symmetrical or asymmetrical
    right side prominent, left side prominent			

Evaluation for Level Pelvis (Figure 4.16) level, tilted to right, tilted to left			
Evaluation of the Knees (Figures 4.17–4.20) come together, stay over feet, splay apart			

Evaluation of Ankle and Foot Alignment
    Heel and Ankle from Behind (right)
    collapses in, straight, collapses out			

Flexibility and Alignment Worksheet

	Date ☞			

Evaluation of Ankle and Foot Alignment (continued)
  Heel and Ankle from Behind (left)
  collapses in, straight, collapses out				

Foot and Toes (right)
  Arch: normal, flat, high
  Big toe: normal, deviates outward
  claw toes, hammer toes				

Foot and Toes (left)
  Arch: normal, flat, high
  Big toe: normal, deviates outward
  claw toes, hammer toes				

Evaluation of Shoulder Flexibility (right) (Figures 4.22, 4.23) normal, limited				
Evaluation of Shoulder Flexibility (left) (Figures 4.22, 4.23) normal, limited				
Evaluation of Hip Flexibility (right) (Figures 4.24, 4.25) normal, limited				
Evaluation of Hip Flexibility (left) (Figures 4.24, 4.25) normal, limited				

Evaluation of Sacroiliac Joint Asymmetry
(Figures 4.26–4.28)
  equal, unequal
  tender on right or left side				

Evaluation of Abdominal Strength (Figures 4.29, 4.30) very weak, moderately weak, moderately strong				

Evaluation of Hamstring Flexibility (Figures 4.31–4.33)
  normal, limited
  distance of buttocks to wall				

Evaluation of Inner Thigh Flexibility (Figures 4.34)
  normal, decreased
  width that legs can spread (in degrees)				

Flexibility and Alignment Worksheet

	Date ☞			
Seated Evaluation of Lumbar Curve (Figures 4.1–4.3) flat, normal, sway				
Standing Evaluation of Lumbar Curve (Figures 4.4–4.6) flat, normal, sway				
Evaluation of Thoracic Curve (Figures 4.7–4.8) increased, normal, decreased				
Evaluation of Right Shoulder Roundedness and Right Shoulder Blade Position (Figures 4.9–4.11) rounded, normal, high, low				
Evaluation of Left Shoulder Roundedness and Left Shoulder Blade Position (Figures 4.9–4.11) rounded, normal, high, low				

Evaluation of Standing Alignment from Side (Figure 4.12)
    Head
    forward, normal, back				

Center of Knee Joint (right) behind ankle, over ankle, in front of ankle				
Center of Knee Joint (left) behind ankle, over ankle, in front of ankle				
Evaluation of Standing Alignment from Back (Figures 4.13, 4.14) spine straight, lateral curves				

Evaluation for Possible Scoliosis (Figure 4.15)
    back ribs symmetrical or asymmetrical
    right side prominent, left side prominent				

Evaluation for Level Pelvis (Figure 4.16) level, tilted to right, tilted to left				
Evaluation of the Knees (Figures 4.17–4.20) come together, stay over feet, splay apart				

Evaluation of Ankle and Foot Alignment
    Heel and Ankle from Behind (right)
    collapses in, straight, collapses out				

Flexibility and Alignment Worksheet

	Date ☞			
Evaluation of Ankle and Foot Alignment (continued) Heel and Ankle from Behind (left) collapses in, straight, collapses out				
Foot and Toes (right) Arch: normal, flat, high Big toe: normal, deviates outward claw toes, hammer toes				
Foot and Toes (left) Arch: normal, flat, high Big toe: normal, deviates outward claw toes, hammer toes				
Evaluation of Shoulder Flexibility (right) (Figures 4.22, 4.23) normal, limited				
Evaluation of Shoulder Flexibility (left) (Figures 4.22, 4.23) normal, limited				
Evaluation of Hip Flexibility (right) (Figures 4.24, 4.25) normal, limited				
Evaluation of Hip Flexibility (left) (Figures 4.24, 4.25) normal, limited				
Evaluation of Sacroiliac Joint Asymmetry (Figures 4.26–4.28) equal, unequal tender on right or left side				
Evaluation of Abdominal Strength (Figures 4.29, 4.30) very weak, moderately weak, moderately strong				
Evaluation of Hamstring Flexibility (Figures 4.31–4.33) normal, limited distance of buttocks to wall				
Evaluation of Inner Thigh Flexibility (Figures 4.34) normal, decreased width that legs can spread (in degrees)				

Glossary

Abdominals. The layers of muscles that form the abdominal wall. These muscles rotate the trunk and bend it forward. They also help maintain the proper tilt of the pelvis and provide additional lumbar support by holding the abdominal contents against the lumbar spine (Figure 2.7).

Activate. To contract several groups of muscles simultaneously in order to stabilize a joint in a position of correct alignment.

Acute. An "acute" disease has a rapid onset, a short duration, and pronounced symptoms. An "acute" pain is sharp or severe.

Adductors. Inner thigh muscles whose action is to move the two thighs toward each other (used to grip the saddle in horseback riding, for example).

Anterior. Toward the front of the body.

Arthritis. A general term meaning inflammation of the joints.

Bolster. A firm pillow used for support in yoga poses. See Resources.

Bone spurs. Bony protrusions usually formed as a result of abnormal forces upon a bone.

Bulging disc. A degenerative condition in which part of the inner substance of an intervertebral disc bulges or protrudes beyond its usual confines (Figure 2.4).

Capillaries. The tiniest blood vessels in the body.

Center of gravity. The balance point of the body, normally located between the navel and the spine.

Cervical. Having to do with the neck.

Chronic. Longstanding, as opposed to acute.

Degenerative disc disease. Changes in the spinal vertebrae and intervertebral discs in which the discs degenerate and become thinner. As a result, the adjacent vertebrae develop structural deformities in an attempt to maintain the spine's ability to absorb shock.

Dysfunction. Impaired functioning.

Disc. An abbreviated term for intervertebral disc.

Eyebag. A cotton or silk bag filled with dry rice that can be placed over the eyes to block out light and enhance relaxation. See Resources.

Facet joints. The flat-surfaced joints between the vertebrae on either side of the spine (Figure 2.3).

Forward head posture. Posture in which, when viewed from the side of the body, the ear hole is in front of the center of the shoulder joint.

Hamstrings. The group of large muscles at the back of the thigh whose main function is to straighten the hip and bend the knee (Figure 2.7).

Herniated disc. A condition in which part of a bulging or degenerated intervertebral disc breaks off. The herniated fragment can press painfully on nerves or the spinal cord.

Hip flexors. The muscles that bend the thigh toward the chest (Figure 2.7).

Hyperextension, hyperextended. A condition in which a joint, such as the knee or the elbow, has been overstraightened past the correct straight alignment (Figure 4.21).

Hypermobile. Capable of abnormally increased movement.

Hypomobile. Incapable of normal movement.

Iliopsoas. Muscles of the hip flexor group that span the space between the upper end of the thigh bone and the inner side of the lumbar spine and the upper pelvis. They can either lift the thigh toward the chest or pull the lumbar spine and pelvis into a swayback (Figure 2.7).

Intervertebral discs. The pads of cartilage that separate the vertebrae (Figure 2.4).

Iyengar-style yoga. A system of yoga developed by B.K.S. Iyengar that emphasizes precise alignment in yoga poses and adaptation of the poses for individual students' needs.

Ligaments. Dense bands of connective tissue (collagen) that connect one bone to another.

Lumbar. Having to do with the lower back or the portion of the spine above the sacrum and below the ribs (Figure 2.1).

Neuromuscular. Having to do with the muscles that move the body and the nerves that coordinate their activity.

Nonskid mat. A thin, relatively noncompressible, nonslippery mat used for yoga practice. See Resources.

Osteoporosis. A condition in which the bones become abnormally porous and easily fractured.

Paraspinals. The bundles of muscles on either side of the spine (Figure 2.6).

Pectorals. Muscles of the upper front chest beneath the breasts. They round the shoulders forward and move the upper arm bone closer to the center of the chest.

Pelvis. The funnel-shaped group of bones that joins the spine to the legs (Figure 2.5).

Piriformis. The muscles that span the space between the sacrum and the upper end of the thigh bone, crossing over the sciatic nerve. The piriformis muscles rotate the thighs outward so the toes point away from the midline of the body (Figure 8.6).

Prepain. The earliest signals that pain is about to occur.

Pubic bone. The front of the pelvis in the midline of the body. If you move your fingers downward from your navel, the first bone you feel will be your pubic bone (Figure 2.5).

Quadriceps. The large group of front thigh muscles that bends the hip and straightens the knee, part of the hip flexor group (Figure 2.7).

Radiating pain. A sharp pain that shoots along the length of a nerve.

Reactive bone changes. A condition in which new bone forms as a result of abnormal stresses.

Relaxation Breath. A simple yoga breathing technique in which you pause for one to three seconds at the end of each normal exhalation, then inhale normally (Chapter 5).

Sacroiliac (SI) joints. The joints on either side of the sacrum where the iliac bones of the pelvis are connected to the sacrum (Figure 2.5). To locate your SI joints, see Figure 4.26.

Sacrum. The triangular bone at the base of the spinal column. The sacrum forms the back of the pelvic funnel (Figure 2.5). To locate your sacrum, see Figure 4.25.

Sciatica. Pain caused by irritation of the sciatic nerve. Sciatica is usually characterized by shooting pain down the back of the leg (Figure 8.6).

Scoliosis. An abnormal side-to-side curvature of the spine (Chapter 10).

Sitting bones. The bony knobs at the base of the pelvis that bear the weight of the body when sitting erect (Figure 2.5).

Spondylolisthesis, spondylolysis. A fracturing of one (spondylolysis) or both (spondylolisthesis) of the connections between adjacent vertebrae. These conditions permit abnormal movement or forward slippage of the spine (Figure 4.35).

Supine. Lying on the back.

Thoracic. Refers to the chest, or the region of the spine where the ribs attach (Figure 2.1).

Thoracic cage. The rib cage.

Torque, torsion. Twisting force.

Total Torso Breathing. Natural breathing in which the muscles of the abdomen and pelvis are relaxed and the chest is allowed to expand (Chapter 6).

Vertebrae. The spool-shaped bones that make up the spine (Figures 2.1, 2.2).

Yoga. The ancient philosophical and therapeutic system developed in India to encourage harmonious living and mental and physical health.

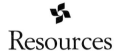

Resources

Yoga Teacher Information

To find out about Iyengar-style yoga, a teacher in your area, and teacher training, contact the following associations.

United States

B.K.S. Iyengar Yoga National Association
   of the United States, Inc.
P.O. Box 79561
Atlanta, GA 30357
800·889·YOGA
http://www.iyoga.com/IYNAUS/

Canada

Canadian Iyengar Yoga
   Teachers Association
c/o 2428 Yonge St.
Toronto, Ont. M4P 2H4
416·482·1333

Books

Relax and Renew
Judith Lasater, Ph.D., P.T. (Berkeley, Calif.: Rodmell Press, 1995)
Practice restorative yoga, supported poses and breathing techniques that ease chronic stress. Includes routines for back pain, menstruation, pregnancy, menopause, and more.

Yoga for Pregnancy
Sandra Jordan (New York: St. Martin's Press, 1987)
A guide to help pregnant women adjust to the demands of labor, birth, and motherhood. Includes 92 Iyengar-style yoga poses, chosen for their safety and effectiveness during and after pregnancy.

The New American Diet
William Connor, M.D., and Sonja Connor, M.S., R.D. (New York: Simon and Schuster, 1990)
The lifetime family diet, based on a major study of American families and funded by The National Institutes of Health, that allows you to lose weight naturally and permanently.

Sex and Back Pain
Lauren Hebert, P.T. (Bangor, Maine:
IMPACC, 1995. Available from IMPACC,
89 Hillside Ave., Bangor ME 04401;
800·762·7720)
An illustrated booklet that shows you how
to adapt your sex life to the needs of your
back.

Magazines/Newsletter

*The Journal of the International Association
    of Yoga Therapists*
(20 Sunnyside Ave., Suite A243, Mill Valley,
CA 94941; 415·332·2478;
http://www.yoganet.com)
Articles, essays, interviews, and book
and video reviews from experts in yoga
therapeutics.

Menopause News
(2074 Union St., San Francisco, CA 94123;
800·241·MENO)
An innovative newsletter with information
on medical facts, alternative therapies,
psychological effects, resources, statistics,
book reviews, and more.

Yoga International
(RR 1, Box 407, Honesdale, PA 18431;
800·253·6243; YImag@epix.net)
Articles and interviews on yoga philosophy,
poses, breathing techniques, meditation,
personal growth, and more. *YI* publishes
an annual *Guide to Yoga Teachers and
Classes*, a supplement to the December/
January issue.

Yoga Journal
(2054 University Ave., Suite 600,
Berkeley, CA 94704; 800·436·9642;
http://www.yogajournal.com)
Body/mind approaches to personal and
spiritual development, such as hatha yoga,
meditation, and more. *YJ* publishes an annual *Directory of Yoga Teachers* in the July/
August issue; also available as a booklet.

Audio

Relaxation
Mary Pullig Schatz, M.D. (Nashville, Tenn.:
Physical Medicine Associates. Distributed
by Rodmell Press, 2147 Blake St.,
Berkeley, CA 94704; 800·841·3123;
RodmellPrs@aol.com)
Soothe body and mind with three guided
relaxation sessions. One tape, 60 minutes,
$9.95, plus $5.00 s/h. Calif. residents add
sales tax.

Yoga Aids, Furniture, and Accessories

Fish Crane
P.O. Box 791029
New Orleans, LA 70179
800·959·6116
Nonskid mats, blankets, and more.

Half Moon Yoga Props
2–2137 W. First Ave., #2
Vancouver, B.C. V6K 1E7
604·731·7099
Blocks, nonskid mats, and more.

Hugger-Mugger Yoga Products
31 W. Gregson Ave.
Salt Lake City, UT 84115
800·473·4888
http://yogacentral.com/hugger
Nonskid mats, blankets, and more.

Iyengar Yoga Bolsters
Capitol Bedding
P.O. Box 1
Baton Rouge, LA 70821
Firm, 100 percent cotton-stuffed and
-covered bolsters for use as yoga props.

Julie Lawrence
600 S.W. Tenth Ave., #406
Portland, OR 97205
i-Ease Eyebag: A rice-filled satin bag to
place over the eyes during relaxation.

Living Arts
2434 Main St., 2nd Floor
Santa Monica, CA 90405
800·2·LIVING
http://www.livingarts.com
This elegant catalog offers a wide selection
of props, clothes, books, tapes, and more.

Rodmell Press Yoga Practice Essentials
2147 Blake St.
Berkeley, CA 94704
800·841·3123
RodmellPrs@aol.com
Eyebags, neck pillows, Savasana pillows,
The Headache Band™, and more.

Tools for Yoga
P.O. Box 99
Chatham, NJ 07928
201·966·5311
Mats, blankets, benches, blocks, belts,
and more.

Yoga Props
731 Florida St.
San Francisco, CA 94110
415·285·YOGA
yogaprops@sfo.com
Wide selection of handcrafted yoga props.

Yogaware
1509 Kearney Rd.
Ann Arbor, MI 48104
313·663·6819
Yoga exercise clothing and props.

Exercise Information and Sources

*American College of Obstetrics
   and Gynecology*
ACOG Resource Center
409 Twelfth St. S.W., P.O Box 96920
Washington, DC 20090–6920
800·762·ACOG
ACOG Home Exercise Programs:
"Exercise During Pregnancy and the
Postpartum Period."

Rockport Walking Institute
220 Donald Lynch Blvd.
Marlboro, MA 01752
508·485·2090
Information on walking physiology, shoes,
walking as a hobby, walking vacations,
walking magazine.

Yoga Vacations

Feathered Pipe Ranch
Box 1682
Helena, MT 59624
406·442·8196
fpranch@initco.net
Offering a variety of week-long residential yoga vacations and other programs, Feathered Pipe Ranch provides opportunities for people to become healthier in body, mind, and spirit.

Bibliography

Chapter 2
Understanding Your Back

Corrigan, B., and G.D. Maitlan. *Practical Orthopedic Medicine*. London: Butterworth, 1983, pp. 237–238.

Gracovetsky, S., et al. "The Importance of Pelvic Tilt On Reducing Compressive Stress in the Spine," *Spine*. 14:412, 1989.

McKenzie, R.A. *The Lumbar Spine: Mechanical Diagnosis and Therapy*. Waikanae, New Zealand: Spinal Publications, Ltd., 1981.

Paris, S.V. *Spinal Dysfunction, Course Notes*. Privately printed, 1979.

Paris, S.V. "Anatomy as Related to Function and Pain," *Orthopedic Clinics of North America*. 14:475, July 1983.

Chapter 3
Moving Again After Injury or Surgery

Arem, A.J., and Madden, J.W. "Effects of Stress on Healing Wounds," *Journal of Surgical Research*. 20:93–102, 1976.

Gordon, R.S. "From the N.I.H.: Sensitivity to Pain," *Journal of the American Medical Association*. 250:18, 1983.

Hepburn, G.R. "Contracture Management," *Journal of Orthopedic and Sports Physical Therapy*. 8:498, 1987.

Holm, S., and Nachemson, A.L. "Nutrition of the Intervertebral Disc: Acute Effects of Cigarette Smoking," *International Journal of Microcirculation Clinical Experimentation*. 3:406, 1984.

Kottke, F., et al. "The Rationale for Prolonged Stretching for Correction of Shortening of Connective Tissue," *Archives of Physical Medicine and Rehabilitation*. 47:345, 1966.

Madden, J.W. "Current Concepts of Wound Healing as Applied to Hand Surgery," *Orthopedic Clinics of North America*. 1:325, November 1970.

Madding, S.W., et al. "Effect of Duration of Passive Stretch on Hip Abduction Range of Motion," *Journal of Orthopedic and Sports Physical Therapy*. 8:409, 1987.

Nachemson, A.L. "Advances in Low Back Pain," *Clinical Orthopedics and Related Research*. 200:266, November, 1985.

Paris, S.V. *Spinal Dysfunction, Course Notes*. Privately printed, 1979.

Chapter 4
Assessing Your Flexibility and Alignment

Kendall, H.O., Kendall, F.P., and Boynton, D.A. *Posture and Pain.* Malibar, Fla.: Robert E. Kreiger Publishing Co., 1975.

Kendall, H.O., Kendall, F.P., and Wadsworth, G.E. *Muscles: Testing and Function.* Baltimore, Md.: Williams and Wilkins, 1971

Chapter 5
Relaxation Techniques

Iyengar, B.K.S. *Light on Yoga.* New York: Schocken, 1979.

Johnson, J.H., and Sarason, I.G. "Life Stress, Depression and Anxiety: Locus of Control as a Moderator Variable," *Journal of Psychosomatic Research.* 22:205, 1978.

Kobasa, S.O., et al. "Hardiness and Health: A Prospective Study," *Journal of Personality and Social Psychology.* 42:168, 1982.

McCaul, K.D., at al. "Effects of Paced Respirations and Expectations on Physiologic and Psychologic Responses to Threat," *Journal of Personality and Social Psychology.* 37:564, 1979.

Selye, H. *The Stress of Life.* New York: McGraw-Hill, 1978.

Wallace, R.K., and Benson, H. "The Physiology of Meditation," *Scientific American.* 226:84, 1972.

Zachariae, R., et al. "Effect of Psychological Intervention in the Form of Relaxation and Guided Imagery on Cellular Immune Function in Normal Healthy Subjects," *Psychotherapy and Psychomatics.* 54:32, 1990.

Chapter 6
Home Base Poses

Iyengar, B.K.S. *Light on Yoga.* New York: Schocken, 1979.

Chapter 7
Moving On Poses

Iyengar, B.K.S. *Light on Yoga.* New York: Schocken, 1979.

Chapter 8
Sacroiliac Pain and Sciatica

Corrigan, B., and Maitlan, G.D. *Practical Orthopedic Medicine.* London: Butterworth, 1983, pp. 258–259, 324.

dePalma, A.F., and Rothman, R.G. *The Intervertebral Disc.* Philadelphia: W.B. Saunders Company, 1970, p. 336.

Iyengar, B.K.S. *Light on Yoga.* New York: Schocken, 1979.

Kendall, H.O., Kendall, F.P., and Boynton, D.A. *Posture and Pain.* Malibar, Fla.: Robert E. Krieger Publishing Company, 1975, pp. 133, 138–141.

Chapter 9
Rounded Upper Back, Forward
Head Posture, and Neck Pain

Iyengar, B.K.S. *Light on Yoga.* New York:
Schocken, 1979.

Chapter 10
Scoliosis

Iyengar, B.K.S. *Light on Yoga.* New York:
Schocken, 1979.

Poussa, M., et al. "Spinal Mobility in Adolescent Girls with Idiopathic Scoliosis,"
Spine. 14:217, 1989.

Chapter 11
A Woman's Back

Iyengar, Geeta S. *Yoga: A Gem for Women.*
Menlo Park, Calif.: Timeless Books, 1990.

Jenkins, S., et al. "Endometriosis: Patho-
genetic Implications of the Anatomic
Distribution," *Obstetrics Gynecology.*
67:335, 1986.

Logue, C.M., and Moos, R.H. "Perimen-
strual Symptoms: Prevalence and Risk
Factors," *Psychosomatic Medicine.*
48:388, July/August, 1986.

Macek, C. "Neurological Deficits: Back
Pain Tied to Endometriosis," *Journal of
the American Medical Association.*
249:686, 1983.

National Institutes of Health, "Consensus
Conference on Osteoporosis," *Journal of
the American Medical Association.*
252:799, 1984.

Chapter 12
Yoga of Daily Living

Nachemson, A. "The Lumbar Spine,"
Spine. 1:81, 1976.

Chapter 13
Exercising Safely

deVries, H.A., et al. "The Tranquilizer
Effect of Exercise," *American Journal of
Physical Medicine.* 61:111, 1982.

Holm, S., and Nachemson, A. "Variations
in Nutrition of Canine Intervertebral
Discs Induced by Motion," *Spine.*
8:866, 1983.

Nachemson, A.L. "Advances in Low Back
Pain," *Clinical Orthopedics and Related
Research.* 200:266, 1985.

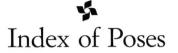

Index of Poses

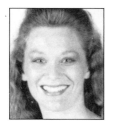

Donna Gurchiek is a registered dietitian and licensed nutritionist. Her special interests include health/wellness and the promotion of positive lifestyles. Donna and her husband, David, became first-time parents on July 20, 1991. Reed Donovan Gurchiek weighed six pounds and six ounces.

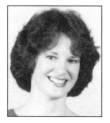

Carol Nelson has been a student and teacher of yoga since 1976, when she first studied with B.K.S. Iyengar. She cofounded and has been the director of the Creative Yoga Studio in Brookline, Massachusetts, for the past twelve years. Along with her yoga practice, Carol enjoys studies in classical music, gardening, and life on the island of Martha's Vineyard.

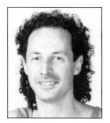

François Raoult has a master's degree in ethnomusicology. He began teaching yoga in 1975 in his native France, where he studied with Noelle Perez-Christiaens and B.K.S. Iyengar. His teaching has been deeply influenced by Ms. Perez-Christiaens's research on yoga and postural alignment. He has also traveled to India many times to study with Iyengar and with his daughter, Geeta. François and his wife, Deborah Granger-Raoult, moved to the United States in 1985 and founded the Center for Aplomb and Yoga in Rochester, New York. Deborah and François have three children.

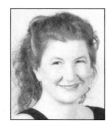

Mary Pullig Schatz, M.D., graduated from Vanderbilt University School of Medicine, where she also completed specialty training in pathology. Dr. Schatz has successfully used yoga to heal her own lower back and neck problems. A certified Iyengar yoga teacher, she teaches yoga to health professionals, medical patients, and other yoga teachers. Correspondence to Dr. Schatz can be addressed to Rodmell Press, 2147 Blake St., Berkeley, CA 94704; RodmellPrs@aol.com.